Parkinson's Disease Battle Manual

Parkinson's Disease Battle Manual

L. E. HEWITT

PUREWAL PUBLISHING, LLC

NOBLESVILLE

Published by
Purewal Publishing, LLC
176 W. Logan Street #105
Noblesville, Indiana 46060-1437
www.SuzannePurewal.com

Cover Design by Suzanne Purewal

Front Cover Image generated with AI by RBGallery, Adobe Stock Photos, AdobeStock_683412462 extended license, Prompt: Man raising hands

Author Photograph by Suzanne Purewal

ISBN: 978-1-7322880-4-1 (print version)

ISBN: 978-1-7322880-5-8 (e-book version)

Library of Congress Card Catalog Number: 2024910174

Printed in the United States of America

I dedicate this book to my fellow Parkinson's brothers and sisters. We fight this battle as one family.

Additional Titles by L. E. Hewitt

Life Between the Raindrops
My Wonderful Chaos
Chasing the Silver Lining
I Don't Have a Button for That
My Bucket List Has a Hole in It
Free TP and Frog Cures
Betty's Best — A Cook's Family Cookbook
Finally! An Unexpected Love Story

Contents

Part II. Common Symptoms

Part III. Things to Consider

Part IV. Fortifying Your Arsenal

Disclaimer

The subject matter in this book is not meant to diagnose, treat, cure, or prevent any disease. It is merely the author's opinions and thoughts on how he has been living and thriving with Parkinson's disease.

There are no implied or guaranteed results. Individual results may vary. The author's views and additional testimonials contained within are not claimed to represent the results you will achieve. All the testimonials are from real people with Parkinson's disease and may not reflect your experience and are not intended to represent or guarantee that anyone will achieve the same or similar results. Each person has unique genetic makeup, exercise habits, eating habits, and responds in a different way. Therefore, the experiences described in this book may not reflect your experience.

The statements, ideas, and recommendations presented in this book are based on the personal experiences, views, and opinions of the author and do not necessarily reflect those of the publisher. They in no way are a substitute for consulting with medical professionals in assessing symptoms and diagnosing and treating any medical condition. Always consult with a medical professional before starting or stopping any treatment, medication, diet, or exercise regimen.

Forward

The *Parkinson's Disease Battle Manual*, written by Lynn Hewitt, is a narrative about an extraordinary middle-aged man who has faced the obstacles, anxiety, and many challenges that come with being diagnosed with Parkinson's disease (PD). Through his journey, Lynn shares many discoveries about himself from which his audience is sure to gain inspiration.

I am honored to have been asked to write a forward for his work and hope to expand on the reasons that this manual is so important for people with Parkinson's disease (PwPD) and why Lynn's perspective is so important for readers, especially folks who are newly diagnosed with PD.

I have been a long-time coach and friend of Lynn's for over six years. I have seen firsthand how he gracefully handles, not just the way he battles his PD, but also how he *chooses* to use optimism and humor to create a better overall quality of life for himself and the people in his life.

My name is Coach K. Rose, and I am one of the founders and long-time coaches of Rock Steady Boxing (RSB). RSB was founded in 2006, in

Indianapolis, Indiana. We now have over 900 RSB affiliate locations in all fifty states and in fourteen different countries.

Our mission is to empower people with PD to fight back with physical fitness and emotional support. The physical fitness modality that RSB uses is a combination of non-contact boxing, martial arts, cardio training, strength training, balance, agility, power movements, and cognitive challenges to help combat many of the symptoms of Parkinson's. Collectively, RSB is serving about 40,000 people with Parkinson's worldwide, and the program has been proven scientifically, through medical research, to slow the progression of PD.

Clinical research has proven that the concept of *intense* exercise, in other words, pushing beyond perceived limits, in addition to a multifunctional style of movement to include strength, rotation, speed of movement, balance, mental focus, and core strength, can *slow* the progression of PD symptoms.

The RSB Method has been tailored to include all these recommendations, in addition to including Parkinson's-specific exercises to address various symptoms of Parkinson's, such as learning proper gait, posture exercises, getting up and down safely from a seated position or floor-to-standing, and even how to fall safely.

In 2021, Rock Steady Boxing was awarded the very first accreditation from The Parkinson Foundation in meeting all standards as an Accredited Exercise Education Program.

While we *know* the physical benefits have been compared to the concept of "exercise is medicine" and works, we also have seen firsthand through almost two decades of the RSB program that "laughter is medicine" through what we call the "fun factor."

Lynn accurately compares this crazy concept of applying a combination of a good medical team, proper medication, and exercise to help in his fight. He further demonstrates through his lifestyle that *laughter* and *fun* play a huge part in maintaining the Parkinson's soul! Lynn is not afraid to push his physical limitations and combat the fear of his own future battling PD. He's also not afraid to make fun of himself and the disease along the way. He acknowledges the importance of finding your PD tribe—an unexpected benefit of fighting back and making the best of a seemingly bad situation.

While some PwPD might allow desperation and despair to creep into their being, Lynn chooses to find unorthodox ways to battle his disease, keep his hands up, and turn adversity into an opportunity.

So proud of you, my friend. You will help many by sharing your story, your heart, and your journey as you continue to fight the good fight.

Don't let what you can't do stop you from what you still can!

Kristy Rose Follmar ACSM, CPT, CIFT

PART I
THE BASICS

In this first part of the book, I detail my journey to reach my Parkinson's diagnosis. Then, I present and discuss what I consider my basic essentials, medical and otherwise, that I utilize in my battle against Parkinson's disease.

1. Introduction

You've been diagnosed with Parkinson's disease. Now what? Of course, there is the initial shock of hearing this news from your doctor. Once you're home, you do Internet searches of all of the horrible things that might or could happen. Then, you wonder how to tell your family, your friends, and your employer.

So many questions to answer. How quickly am I going to decline? Is someone gonna need to take care of me? Feed me? Bathe me? Worse? Am I gonna die soon? Do I need to get my affairs in order? Why me? How did I get this? Where did it come from?

Yes, the questions are nearly endless at first. This may be the most significant thing you have ever faced, and it's incurable and degenerative. It can be overwhelming. It would be easy to go home, turn on the television, sit in the recliner, and wait to die. Why not? Can't be cured, gonna get worse, uncontrollable tremors, dementia, hallucinations, rigidity, this just sounds horrible! Plus, you've now read through half a dozen websites, and there is nothing but doom and gloom ahead.

Well, gee, that's not exactly what you wanted to read about today, is it? It's okay, nearly every person with a Parkinson's disease (PD) diagnosis mourns for themselves at first. An unwelcome guest has entered your world, and it never plans to leave.

Contrary to what you're thinking, it is not the end of the world. What I hope to accomplish with this book is to share my Parkinson's journey with you to help you better understand ways to cope, battle, and hopefully improve your current outlook and quality of life.

2. My Story

Let me tell you a little about me. I'm a sixty-one-year-old man who lives in the midwestern United States. I was a relatively healthy average guy, nothing significant to report until age forty-seven. That's when I suffered a mild stroke. It was really a shock. I never had major health concerns prior to this event.

I arrived home late one evening from my job. At the time, the job was stressful, as was my home life. I felt overwhelmed and tired. It was around 10:00 P.M. when I went downstairs to use the home computer. After a few minutes, I discovered that my right hand didn't want to function correctly. I was having difficulty controlling the mouse to navigate the cursor. My fingers felt clumsy. I shook them around a little and wrote it off to maybe a bit of carpal tunnel or something similar and went to bed.

The following morning, my hand still felt odd, my arm felt numb, and I was mentally sluggish. I didn't experience any particularly acute symptoms. They were more subtle than anything. However, it was concerning enough for me to call my primary care physician (PCP).

Fortunately, my PCP was the type of guy who was readily available to his patients. We had an immediate chat on the telephone. He agreed with me that it was probably nothing of significant concern for a healthy man in his late forties. But, to be safe, I should come on over to the office to see him. His office was a ten-minute drive away, so off I went.

Upon arriving, my doctor checked all the usual stuff—blood pressure, reflexes, and temperature. Additionally, he had me do a few other minor things. After these standard checks, he stood there before me scratching his head. He was perplexed. Something was off. But was this just a minor mystery or something more significant beginning to appear? He sent me over to the hospital for an MRI of my brain as a precaution.

My unplanned morning was expanding into new territory. I arrived for the STAT MRI and was quickly slid into that magic, noisy cylinder. Waiting for results didn't take long. Shortly thereafter, my doctor called to inform me that, much to his own surprise, I had suffered a stroke!

At first, the scary part was that the doctor didn't know the root cause or if this was a precursor to a bigger stroke. I was literally living in uncertainty. I didn't like that feeling at all.

I endured a whole myriad of tests. They showed I was basically healthy, but a blood clot had formed. In the end, my ongoing treatment consisted of a blood pressure pill and an aspirin each day.

The neurologist later told me that my chances of having another stroke were only negligibly higher than an average person, simply because I'd previously had an event. The only telltale sign of a past stroke was a lacuna (a small dead space) in my brain.

It took me about six months to return to relatively normal function, and I continued to see my neurologist regularly for monitoring, but my life went forward.

In retrospect, the stroke was the best thing that ever happened to me. On the surface, that proclamation doesn't sound very logical, does it? Well, let me explain. Prior to the stroke, I was like the majority of adults, constantly stressed about bills, work, children, my own mortality, the health of my aging parents, mistakes I'd made in the past, what was going to happen tomorrow, my goals for next year, and my plan for my retirement. Stress, stress, followed by even more stress, rarely living in the moment.

When I first had the stroke, I didn't know if I would even have a tomorrow to worry about, and suddenly, past mistakes were unimportant. All that mattered was right now, this minute, nothing else.

How could I make the most of now for myself, my children, my life? I genuinely started living in the present. I strived to make each day a celebration and to make every moment as good as it could be. Then, something totally unexpected happened. By living in the present, I became happy, *genuinely* happy from within. Every day became filled with absolute joy. I came to realize what a blessing each day could be, and that yesterday and tomorrow were far less important than right now. All of my stress melted away. I was literally transformed. My only regret was that it had taken me almost fifty years to have this epiphany.

Unfortunately, I have found that this perspective is very difficult to teach others. We are all so conditioned by society to be constantly rushing to the next project, the next holiday, the next job, or the next chore. People have a difficult time trying to focus on the present.

Of course, I do encounter others who are like me. They just know what I am talking about, and you can even see genuine joy in their smiles. Many of these people have also faced some sort of life crisis which helped transform them.

I know, I've talked about all sorts of things besides Parkinson's disease. My apologies, but I'm getting there.

A few years passed after the stroke. I was doing reasonably well, yet I developed some lingering symptoms that perplexed my neurologist. I felt off balance. I would be walking on a perfectly smooth concrete floor and feel as if I were on the side of a hill. I would sometimes stumble, often not forward or backward, but sideways, due to this sensation. Some days, I felt completely exhausted. It was overwhelming to even get up out of the chair to go to the bathroom or the mailbox or do any basic household chore.

I would get funky sensations I described as brain jolts. They felt sort of like an electrical shock being sent through my head, just a quick zap. I could feel one coming a couple of seconds before it would occur. The zaps were not what I would describe as painful. They were more like an interruption in my normal circuitry.

My short-term memory wasn't so great. I experienced difficulty learning new things. For instance, if I had an appointment in the afternoon and was thinking about it in the morning, by the time afternoon arrived, I would forget to go. Occasionally, I forgot food on the stove. Other times, I left water running in the sink. I had never experienced these lapses before, so I had no clue as to what was happening. Some might describe it as brain fog. I simply wasn't thinking clearly. Was this just aging? Just leftover symptoms from the stroke?

The neurologist kept saying something else was going on, and so he kept running tests. I had an EEG, EKG, ENG, and MRI, among others. I think we covered the acronym alphabet. I was subjected to memory testing and the 72-hour brain scan where they hook up 10,000 wires to your head and then send you home. That was highly entertaining at the grocery store. People looked at me like I was highly contagious or a space alien. I also recall a woman who was having a yard sale. I love yard sales and didn't think about my appearance with all of the wires. She had a distressed look, and her two small children apparently thought I was some sort of monster. She sent them into the house when they started crying.

The doctor kept evaluating my brain and nerve functions. Additionally, he conducted the test where they blow air into your ears to try and make you dizzy—it worked! The flood of hot and cold air made everything in the room spin. All I could do was hang onto my pillow for dear life, until things calmed back down.

The neurologist checked for seizures and tumors

and considered several other diseases. He seemed especially focused on my symptoms being some sort of seizure disorder. Yet, the brain function tests didn't show anything significant on that front. Finally, he arrived at the conclusion that I had Parkinson's disease.

There is no definitive test to prove PD, aside from an autopsy, and I wasn't submitting to that! There are tests that can give clues, such as a DaTscan, brainwave testing, nerve conduction testing, and physical testing to gauge gait, balance, and memory function. In the end, it is still a clinical diagnosis, which basically means that it is based upon the observations and conclusions of the doctor.

I have learned in the years since, many people spend a long time seeking a diagnosis. They endure a slew of tests and are even diagnosed with other conditions, sometimes multiple times, before receiving an accurate assessment.

I consider myself fortunate that I was already seeing a specialist regularly for my previous stroke. However, even with that, it still took him a few years to unravel the mystery. The diagnosis path seems to be especially challenging in younger patients. Many doctors simply think of PD as an old person's disease. They are apt to look in other directions first before reaching the correct conclusion.

I still remember that day. It was eight and a half years ago. My doctor walked into the room and said, "I've finally reached the conclusion that you have Parkinson's. Do you have questions for me?"

Well, of course I had questions, but I also told him I would need to familiarize myself with this disease and learn better questions to ask.

As for this being devastating news, well, that's where my previous experience with a stroke came in handy. I already possessed some valuable tools to deal emotionally with bad news. For many people, this will be the worst news they've ever been given. I viewed it as a new challenge, but one I was prepared to face.

I didn't really have much knowledge about PD. I knew of a few people who had it, elderly folks with shaky hands. But, they weren't people I knew well. The only family member who was diagnosed with it was my late father, at the age of eighty-six years old. The doctor told him not to worry about it because it would never be a significant issue in his lifetime. The doctor was correct. My father passed away at eighty-eight years old, of unrelated issues associated with aging. I did recall that he would be amused when his finger or hand would occasionally tremor. It was minor and never of any concern. But, here I was, fifty-two years old, and I had no clue what this was going to do to me. So, like most people, I went home and surfed the Internet.

The first question was, "Is this gonna shorten my life expectancy?" That was the top concern. I quickly discovered that the most basic answer was, "No." Data suggested that life expectancies were typically only minimally impacted. I learned that quality of life was the most significant concern. Often, people didn't die *from* Parkinson's, but instead, they died *with* Parkinson's.

Then, I learned that there are many different types of symptoms that you can get, and that each one of us seems to get our own unique package of challenges. Some get tremors, some do not, some get dementia, some not. Many experience hallucinations, rigidity, or have a weak voice. Others face freezing episodes or pain. The list is very extensive.

In my case, I have body tremors, tongue tremors, occasional balance issues, and short-term memory issues. Certain days, I am totally and completely exhausted.

I do want to tell you to be careful searching the Internet. The answers you find may be confusing. Everything from life expectancies to quality of life issues, to options for treatment, exercise programs, symptoms—everything is different based upon your individual circumstances. A Parkinson's diagnosis for my eighty-six-year-old father was very different than a Parkinson's diagnosis for me at fifty-two years old.

Let me take a sidebar here for a moment. I want you to know that I am not a medical professional. I am not trained in any therapies or treatments. I am simply an expert in my own personal life experiences I've had with my PD journey. There are many resources available from people with years of formal education and training. I'm sharing what I have learned from living with Parkinson's. So, please remember, I do not know everything. I just know me and what's effective for me. You will experience your own mix of symptoms. You might find that some of the treatments and actions that work for me may or may not be beneficial to you. But, we can learn from one another.

A huge consideration with this disease has to do with your own individual age and physical condition at the time of diagnosis. While Parkinson's can be the reason for a variety of afflictions, do not blame every ailment that comes along on your PD. We can still get arthritis, the flu, cancer, heart disease, or any other conditions the average person may encounter. When a new symptom appears, get it checked out.

That's one very large lesson to learn. Your medical team needs to be a regular part of your life from now on. They are a vital link in keeping you healthy and productive for a long time to come.

That's a basic overview of me. The rest of the book will address some essential topics that I believe can help you to have a successful life after diagnosis. At the end of each section, I will ask you to consider how the particular topic relates to you.

Your Battle Plan

1) Did you have any difficulty in finding a diagnosis?

2) How were you affected emotionally by this news?

3) How are you dealing with it now?

4) How were your family/friends/loved ones affected by this news?

5) Have you accepted the challenges Parkinson's presents?

6) Are you ready to meet these challenges head on?

7) Do you have a support system? Consider friends, loved ones, support groups, and/or counseling.

3. Pity Party

Yes, you have Parkinson's disease, and it is here to stay. That's a good reason to mourn. Grief and denial are normal parts of the process. But, you must accept the situation and push on. You must get back in gear and begin living again. You cannot control what has happened. You *can* control how you respond. Yes, you are going to die, someday. You have known that for nearly your whole life. Yes, your health will probably decline as you age. You've known that your whole life too. It is true for almost all of us. Only a few will go from perfect health to death in an instant. I do not desire to be one of them. Getting hit by a truck while crossing the road is not how I want to exit my life.

You've got this big, bad, horrible diagnosis. So, what are you gonna do about it? You have options. You can live in denial and try to ignore it, hide your eyes from the truth, and pretend it doesn't exist. Ignoring a problem is seldom a lasting solution, but you can try.

You can also have a big pity party. You can feel sorry for yourself and convince yourself that life is suddenly over. You can attempt to drown it with alcohol or distract your attention by staring at a television all day. You may even choose to stay in bed and sleep all the time to avoid the emotional pain. Parkinson's disease wants you to do just that. When you do nothing, Parkinson's wins. It is that simple.

For a moment, let's forget about the PD diagnosis and look at life in general. Have you ever contemplated the sheer miracle of your existence? Maybe your life has been great to this point, or maybe not so much. Either way, you are here now because literally billions of events happened in exactly the correct order in your past, which brought every molecule of you together, at exactly the right time in the right place. Otherwise, there would be no you. You would have never lived at all. To me, that's quite incredible. Shouldn't we go ahead and make the most of the opportunity? That is my view at least. I personally feel I should celebrate my good fortune, even on the bad days.

Another miracle is that you exist in a time where the medical sciences can offer you a variety of treatments and therapies for a better quality of life. As little as one hundred years ago, the average life expectancy was only fifty-four years old.

You can choose to focus on your problems and feel sorry for yourself, or you can treat every day as a reason to celebrate because you have already won the life lottery. You are here. You are the winner.

Let's apply these thoughts to Parkinson's. Yes, it is a degenerative disease that will present you with additional challenges. But, you are living in a time where you are equipped with tools that you can utilize to maintain your quality of life. All you need to do is to pick up these tools and use them! What can possibly be the harm in trying? You can do this. You can make the rest of your life better for yourself, and those you love, by utilizing all of the resources available to you. Do not stop. Do not quit. You are already a winner. This is your opportunity to act like one, and show Parkinson's disease that you will not give in. Now, go out there starting immediately, and win that battle every day.

Your Battle Plan

1) Do you find yourself getting down or depressed?

2) What do you do when you're feeling down?

3) Do you have someone to talk to about how you're feeling? If not, are you ready to reach out to someone today?

4) Do you know where to find mental health resources? If not, ask your doctor or get on the Internet and find resources near you.

4. Your Medical Team

You've probably heard the phrase, "It takes a village." With Parkinson's, this is certainly a true concept. Achieving the best quality of life after diagnosis requires the contributions of many skilled individuals, often working together. You quickly learn that you need to be open to utilizing assistance, no matter how independent you may have been to this point.

It's important to remember that this is based upon my personal experiences, so your care team may look very different from mine. The key is to actively pursue and find what works for you. Never just live with a particular problem without first actively seeking a solution. Then, if you have exhausted every option, only then should you identify a workable adaptation. In other words, do not give PD an inch of leverage voluntarily. Fight for every ability it tries to take away. You will be surprised at how often you will win. My personal motto is that I keep dragging my Parkinson's along, and I dare it to keep up with me.

Of course, your care team will include your primary care physician (PCP) because you are still gonna get the flu or allergies or injure yourself from time to time, just like anyone else. It is particularly important to keep other ailments at bay for as long as possible. High blood pressure, diabetes, weight management, depression, anxiety, and a thousand other common maladies are much better controlled with regular medical intervention. Your PCP will remain your first contact for these types of things. I personally see mine about twice a year, unless I have a specific need for additional assistance.

Let me offer a good example. A few months ago, I went to visit my PCP for a swallowing issue. Was this a Parkinson's related problem? Well, maybe, but maybe not. The bottom line—it was something that needed investigation.

I'd noticed certain foods would get stuck in my esophagus on the journey to my stomach. At first, it appeared as an occasional inconvenience, but it progressed and became more frequent and severe. I sought help due to an episode with a chicken sandwich in a fast food joint one afternoon. The food got significantly stuck halfway down. I could breathe, but it was quite painful. I tried coughing, drinking water, and sort of a self-Heimlich, and nothing worked. Finally, after about three minutes, I was able to get it to move enough to resolve the immediate problem. I basically gagged up the lodged water-soaked bread and chicken. It wasn't pretty or fun. It also ruined my desire to eat much for the remainder of the day. My esophagus was sore for a few days from that very unnerving experience.

I contacted my PCP and paid him a visit. He did a brief examination and referred me to a specialist in gastroenterology who scheduled me, on an expedited basis, for an endoscopy.

In case you are not familiar with an endoscopy, it is an easy procedure as a patient. You do not eat or drink for several hours before the procedure. They give you an IV with a marvelous drug that gives you the best sleep you've had since you were a teenager. After you're knocked out, they snake a camera down to and through your stomach and into your small intestines. In my case, they discovered a narrowing in my esophagus. So, they used a balloon-type device to gently stretch and widen that area.

When I awoke, all I noticed was the sensation similar to minor muscle soreness down inside my chest. I avoided hard or sharp foods for a few days. That was it. The end result was amazing. Nothing gets stuck now! It just flies on through with zero problems. I had not realized how much this had been affecting my daily life until it was gone. I noticed that I avoided certain foods and expected discomfort when swallowing others. I hadn't really noticed this until that negative sensation disappeared.

To offer another perspective, one of my friends with Parkinson's also developed a swallowing issue at about the same time as me. His particular circumstance was vastly improved by swallowing exercises given to him by a therapist. I believe his challenge was more of an incomplete swallowing issue rather than a narrowing one like mine. But, the point is that we both had an issue that needed medical intervention. Unnecessary discomfort or decreased quality of life, not to mention the potential for more serious complications, would have continued had we not sought treatment.

Physical and occupational therapists can be invaluable resources for someone with PD. They can assist with balance, strength, proper physical safety measures, and recommend specific tools that can make your life easier. You will discover that these specialists are going to be great assets as you move forward with PD.

You may wonder what sort of tools can be beneficial. I just had a conversation yesterday with someone regarding this type of matter. They were talking about a loved one who struggled to eat without making a mess, due to tremors. They were unaware that weighted utensils could help with this challenge.

Occupational therapists can advise you about all sorts of equipment to improve your daily living. With Parkinson's, you may discover the need for walking aids or adaptations to your bath or shower. You may need to be more selective in buying shoes that provide better support. You may even need to utilize alarms or timers to remember to take medications or to take a pot off of the stove. Due to physically acting out my dreams, I added a small bed rail to my bed.

See, I get off on tangents. I speak of one thing and that leads to another and another and before you know it, I am way off of the original subject. But, that's okay. We will eventually get back to the topic at hand. This is what some of us refer to as "Parkie brain." Our thought processes do not always follow traditional paths. We are often still highly functional, we just bounce around between ideas more frequently.

The next professional in your new PD life will be either a neurologist or a movement disorders specialist. This person will be the one to rely upon to handle PD specific issues and your ongoing treatment.

I've seen my neurologist probably an average of once every three months for over a decade. He tracks my progression with various testing of my brain function, nerve function, balance, agility, and memory. In my case, I get flare-ups of nerve pain. My neurologist has been very effective in treating those issues with trigger point injections. I feel fortunate that he is a caring fellow. He even made time to meet my chiropractor for lunch, so they could coordinate my care. I realize that not all doctors will go that far. So, I feel quite lucky. He will frequently wish to just have a chat and discuss any new or changing symptoms.

My advice is to not hold back when talking to your doctors. Tell them everything. They cannot know many of your specific symptoms unless you share the details with them. These professionals are here to help you. They have dedicated their entire adult lives to being knowledgeable about these conditions. If you hide details from them, you will only be harming yourself.

Yes, I mentioned my chiropractor. Posture is a big deal with PD. We tend to want to hunch over or hang our heads, slouch, and shuffle. My chiropractor keeps my spine in proper alignment and gives me posture exercises. She is also involved in pain management and keeping me comfortable. I have found her services to be well worthwhile. I do not need to see her as regularly, unless I am having an acute issue, but a checkup here and there is still a good idea.

Have you ever been to a chiropractor? It can be a noisy experience with all of those joints popping back into alignment, but I have never experienced any pain from treatment. I have, however, walked into the office in pain and walked out feeling fabulous. She twists me up like a pretzel. She even uses a little gun, an activator, to shoot the tissues at or around my joints. She uses that, along with pressure, to manipulate my joints to realign my spine. The cracking noises are from the trapped gases in the joints being released, similar to cracking your knuckles. I usually walk out feeling refreshed and more fluid in my movements.

Another member of my care team is the acupuncturist. This is possibly someone you may not have considered. Well, let me tell you that for me, she is essential. How do I begin to explain the sensation? I lie down, and she asks me what is hurting. Then, she places several fine needles into various parts of my body. Trust me, it's painless. Once I'm loaded up like a pin cushion, she leaves me alone to take a nap. I drift off into this trancelike sleep. I can literally feel the energy flowing through my body. It is difficult to describe the sensation. But, after maybe forty minutes or so, I awaken. Like a slice of bread popping up out of a toaster, I am fully awake, refreshed, and energized. Then, she removes the needles, and I exit feeling absolutely amazing. I do not understand it. I do not have any clue why or how it works, but for me, it does. Acupuncturists treat anything from migraines to joint pain to neuropathy to fibromyalgia. I go mostly for my nerve pain.

How do I describe my nerve pain? One area I have experienced this malady, on multiple occasions, is around my ribcage. It begins at my spine and radiates all the way around one side of my ribs to the front. It is a sensitivity type of pain. If I slap the area, it doesn't hurt. Yet, my shirt rubbing against it is very uncomfortable. Nerve pain makes it difficult to sleep and uncomfortable to move—nagging, annoying, unrelenting. I've had episodes over the years in my legs, my neck and head, and even my buttocks. I have tried numerous medications and therapies, but for me, acupuncture is one of the most effective treatments for these flare-ups. Remember, you may respond well to medications or more traditional therapies. Our bodies all react differently to various treatments. This is why if one avenue is not successful for you, keep trying until you find what works.

The final member of my own personal medical care team is my massage therapist. Parkinson's disease is filled with rigidity and lack of mobility, muscle tension, and fatigue. A good massage on a regular basis will do wonders to help keep things loosened up. Plus, it's just so darned enjoyable! I try to go monthly. It seems beneficial to both my body and my spirit. Releasing tension and stress on particular areas of my body is money well spent.

Yes, the overall massage experience is enjoyable, but I also know when she finds a "spot." I don't even need to tell her. She will identify an area of tension and attack it. I cannot hide it from her. She just knows. My worst area for these tension knots is in those large muscles that run from my shoulders up the back of my neck. Those get very tight on me. My massage therapist works those out and alleviates the tension. It can be a bit uncomfortable during the process, but it feels so much better once she has alleviated the problem. Of course, she works on my entire body, but in my case, my darned neck is the most challenging area.

That's my personal medical team. Your team may

end up looking quite different, and that's okay. The key is to not do it alone. Or worse yet, do nothing. The fastest route to a bad outcome with PD is to simply go home and remain idle. That will allow the disease to dictate your life, and it will win.

Parkinson's is not managed without a fight. You must be proactive and utilize all of the resources at your disposal. Fortunately, if you do fight for maintaining a better quality of life, the rewards can be immense. The successes may even surprise you. I've seen it in my own life, and I've also witnessed it in others. This diagnosis is not necessarily the end of anything. You may require some adaptations. You may need to work harder than you've ever worked. But, so many people are finding their best lives with PD. Never stop fighting for it.

Your Battle Plan

1) What nagging ailments have you been dealing with?

2) What medical professional(s) do you need to contact today to make an appointment?

3) Which symptom would you most like to improve,

and what is a first step you can take to help make this better?

5. Breaking the News

Breaking the news to the important people in your life is necessary. You might be hesitant. Mostly likely, you are still trying to wrap your head around the idea of having Parkinson's disease. You might be in disbelief. Understandably, you might also be angry, depressed, or in denial. However, the bottom line remains that you have to share your diagnosis. Telling others can seem daunting but the people in your life need to know.

Family is probably the easiest group of people to inform about your diagnosis. Primarily, they are going to be concerned about how this will affect you in the future. They can read on the Internet about it, but it is imperative for them to hear directly from you that you are doing okay, and this is not a death sentence. Talk openly with them about your expectations and the things you have learned about your condition. Explain your specific symptoms and give them the opportunity to understand and empathize with you. Be open when you are having an "off" day or experiencing various symptoms. Remember, they cannot always tell by looking at you. You must share things thoroughly, so they understand.

This next point is HUGE! You need to forever keep this in mind. I have heard far too many stories over the years about PwPD being verbally or physically abusive with their caregivers or other loved ones. I assume this results from frustration and fear. I get that. However, your disease should never ever be an excuse to mistreat those who are trying to help you. *Never.* Do not become that person. Do not allow yourself to misdirect those emotions and hurt those around you.

I do understand that in some cases, due to dementia, hallucinations, or confusion, a person may lash out because they have lost control of their mental faculties. At that point, additional medications or alternate living arrangements may be necessary. I'm not speaking about those situations. I am talking about a deliberate choice to take out your anger or fear on a loved one. That is *never* acceptable.

On the opposite end of the spectrum, do not let your family baby you or tend to your every need. As much as possible, get up and do tasks yourself. Remaining engaged in activities of daily living will serve you well. Whatever your circumstances, do your best to not permit PD to dictate your life and how you live it.

You might be nervous about sharing the news at your workplace. Many people with Parkinson's disease still work. Some work full-time, others may switch to part-time. You may require specific accommodations because of the effects of the disease. Due to balance difficulties and rigidity, there might be a handful of tasks you can no longer safely perform. However, most employers will work with you to modify the tasks of your current position or identify other areas of opportunity in which you are more suited. If you meet resistance, the Americans with Disabilities Act (ADA) is a federal civil rights law that applies to companies with fifteen or more employees. It prohibits discrimination based on disability.

Speaking of disability, I am not sure how it may work in other countries, but here in America, you will possibly qualify for disability benefits due to your Parkinson's diagnosis. This can be a godsend to provide some financial support as you take on this new challenge. It is a drawn-out process, but it can be worthwhile to pursue, if working becomes too difficult.

You've told your family. You've told your boss.

Now, let's discuss your friends. It is somewhat normal that fair-weather friends may drift away during this time. You cannot control that. It's just a reality. Not everyone can handle adversity well. On the flip side, you will have friends who become more engaged, out of concern and caring. Open communication with your friends is big. They may not know that you want to continue playing golf on Thursdays. They might be afraid to bring up the subject, in the event you aren't able to play anymore. Therefore, it is up to you to inform them about your expectations and limitations. Your responsibility is to communicate what is possible. They won't know unless you share openly and honestly.

Twenty-five years ago, one of my golfing buddies was diagnosed with pancreatic cancer. He was given an expectation of a few months to live. My immediate reaction was to assume he was getting his affairs in order and preparing to die. Well, at his urging, for the next several months, he continued to join our group to play golf every week. He did great. Sure, he got fatigued more easily, but he kept right on living and enjoyed his time more because he spoke up and wanted to be there. If he had not advocated for himself, we would have never known. I am glad we shared those extra memories that summer. It was also a few hours when he wasn't focused on his cancer. He was just having fun with friends.

I mentioned that you will have friends who won't be around as much because they cannot deal with your situation. Don't fret over it. You cannot fix that. Make every effort to keep involved with the friends who do stick around. You will find a whole flock of new friends from your Parkinson's activities. If you get involved, you won't be lonely.

Your Battle Plan

1) Are you sharing your situation with everyone who is important to you?

2) Are you communicating your concerns and how you are feeling with them?

3) Are you being kind to loved ones?

4) What sort of adaptations or modifications would be needed for you to continue your current job?

5) What alternative positions might you be better suited?

6. Exercise

I know, I know. Exercise may sound like a dirty word to some folks. Or, you may even say, "I'm too old," or "I've got a bad knee or hip or shoulder," or "I have too many health issues." I've heard them all. That's a knee-jerk response. I find it is often based in fear, incorrect information, stubbornness, or just a general lack of knowledge. The truth is that very few people truly cannot exercise. A number of people won't want to hear that, but it is true, and I will attempt to explain myself.

Again, remember, I have no special degrees or training, but I have observed some amazing things. You see, we all want a magic cure for Parkinson's. It would be nice if the doctor said, "Take this pill once a day, and your Parkinson's will be all gone in a week." That does not exist yet. However, vigorous exercise does do magical things to retain function and slow the progression. Heck, in some cases, I'd be of the opinion that it even reverses progression of the disease, but that's just my layman's opinion.

I said that exercise is for virtually everyone. A qualified physical trainer or coach can demonstrate how to modify any exercise to adapt to your individual circumstances. As an example, an old-fashioned push-up can be done on your hands and toes on the floor. Want it easier? Do it from your hands and knees. Easier? Elevate your hands by using a chair or other sturdy object. Easier? Do your push-ups against a wall. Exercises can be adapted all the way down to wheelchair users and bedridden individuals. Want it harder? Put a clap in between each push-up or only use one arm or one leg.

The key to successful fitness is to begin at your current level and incrementally work to improve. It's that simple. You may amaze yourself. I know individuals who could barely walk in their forties and now run sprints. A guy in his late seventies, who was never into exercise, now runs marathons. Seventy-year-old ladies are doing chin-ups. These are all people with Parkinson's disease. These individuals have chosen to fight for their quality of life.

I am sixty-one years old and more fit than most people half my age. This was not true prior to my diagnosis. I participate in a boxing exercise program designed specifically for Parkinson's patients. Thanks to that program, I run, jump rope, do push-ups, sit-ups, and get down on the floor and stand back up with ease. I am strong. My balance has vastly improved. I easily stand on one leg while putting on my pants.

Ten years ago, I would never have imagined I'd be this physically fit. In addition to my boxing program, I am an avid cyclist. For balance safety, I ride a Tadpole recumbent three-wheel bike. Beginning each spring, I ride a few miles, multiple days per week. I gradually increase my time and distance when training for cycling trips I take with friends. We have made multiple treks on the Great Allegheny Passage and C&O Towpath, a 338-mile ride from Pittsburgh, Pennsylvania to Washington, D.C., through the Appalachian Mountains. It takes us about a week. It is a breathtakingly beautiful trip through nature, plus we get to meet some interesting people along the way. The exercise and camaraderie are good for my body and my spirit.

This year, we are planning a cycling trip through Nova Scotia, for another unique adventure. The cycling is a strenuous cardiovascular workout, plus my legs are kept super strong by this exercise.

I do realize that we are all at different points in our lives, but do not be afraid to push yourself. Whether it's riding around the neighborhood, spending time at home on a stationary bike, or using stationary pedal equipment that you do from a chair, don't give in to PD telling you that you can't. Do not be afraid to challenge yourself and dream big.

Another activity that excites me is racquetball. I enjoy the challenge of the competition. What is nice about racquetball is that younger and older people compete against one another equally. The younger players are quicker, but the older players are typically more effective shot makers. Of course, other similar sports include tennis and pickleball. I know several people with Parkinson's who have taken up pickleball in recent years. I have a friend with PD who travels all over the country competing in pickleball tournaments. He is an inspiration for not allowing his diagnosis to interfere with his goals.

An additional physical exercise regimen is yoga. I have found that it is highly complimentary to my other activities. My yoga sessions increase my strength, balance, and flexibility significantly. The instructor conducts sessions outdoors, in the park, when weather permits. Retaining flexibility is a major part of my battle with PD. Yoga involves slow movements that work your muscles. It is highly adaptable to each individual's abilities. A somewhat similar program that is utilized by many with Parkinson's is Tai Chi.

I do not expect you to follow my exercise routines. I want you to develop a system that works for you.

There are Parkinson's programs that include stretching, strength training, dancing, vocal strengthening, weight training, and swimming. I even joined a group last summer that ran an obstacle course. One fella I know competed on a televised obstacle course competition, in spite of his PD.

The bottom line is to remain active, keep moving, keep living. These types of activities will slow the disease's progression and help you maintain a higher quality of life. Age doesn't matter. I have friends with PD from their thirties to their nineties. There have been occasions when I was running during a workout and was passed by a person, in their mid-eighties, who was diagnosed over twenty years ago. Those moments push me to try harder.

Do not get discouraged by all of this information I am throwing at you. Begin where you are. If that's doing ten arm curls using a soup can, then that is where you begin. Once you have established a baseline, then work to improve. Yes, I may be proposing some lofty goals. I have some of those for myself as well. Keep in mind that you will never achieve anything you do not attempt. Delete the phrase, "I can't," from your vocabulary. Replace it with, "I'm going to find a way."

While we are on the subject of exercise, there is one

crucial area we need to address. This is an essential part of your Parkinson's journey. You absolutely must exercise your brain. Slowing of brain function, dementia, hallucinations, anxiety, and depression can all be associated with this disease. The best way to combat these issues is to keep your brain strong. You've got to keep using that noggin. Challenge yourself to learn new skills and sharpen old ones.

I utilize brain puzzle books I purchase online. I am a musician, so I continue to learn new songs, new skills, and even new instruments. I assemble puzzles and play board games. I play Scrabble against strangers online. These things assist in keeping my brain as healthy as possible. Some things may not be as easy as they once were, and that can be extremely frustrating at times. Do not focus on what you cannot do. Instead, look at all of the things you still can do. You just might be surprised.

I know, I keep using that word, "surprised." That's because I have surprised myself many times over these past several years.

You are still capable of so much! Make use of those skills. You may have a passion for cooking, painting, gardening, or travel. Whatever it is, find a way to make it possible for you. Adaptations may be necessary, but that's okay. Go for it.

In my younger years, I was a professional musician, a drummer. No, I cannot play as well as I once did. Yes, that bothered me at first. In time, I considered it a new challenge. I made various changes to adjust to my current abilities. I do still play on my drum set some. I also added new percussion instruments to my collection—bongos, a cajón, and a djembe. All three instruments are played with my bare hands. These are adaptations that allow me to continue to enjoy my craft.

Constant learning is very satisfying and good for my brain and my body. I've been learning to play the banjo. It's not easy for me. However, I love a good challenge. This instrument requires significant finger picking and totally different chords from a standard guitar. This forces my brain to create new neural pathways, as I learn new skills and attempt to improve my abilities. These hobbies work for me because I have a history with music.

You can discover your own passions. I know PwPD who are playing the cello, designing projects with a 3D printer, getting involved in PD awareness as public speakers and event organizers, working via the Internet as a tutor, teaching grandchildren important life lessons, growing the best vegetable gardens, and writing autobiographies—the list is nearly endless.

Life doesn't stop with a diagnosis. You have to fight and take control of your circumstances.

One of the difficult things about giving advice for living with Parkinson's is that you may be diagnosed at thirty or at ninety. One answer does not fit everyone. However, medical care, exercise, a clean diet, and remaining as engaged as possible are important for every one of us.

I want to briefly cover other types of exercise equipment you may find useful. Many of these items are inexpensive. I personally have a heavy boxing bag, a speed bag, a double-ended bag, a weight bench, a Total Gym, a weighted medicine ball, a stationary recumbent bike, an exercise ball, a BOSU ball, resistance bands, a pull-up bar, and various hand weights. Yes, I've got a stocked gym in my basement. That wasn't always the case. I've used soup cans, water jugs, and my own body weight along with a plain, ordinary chair to do many workouts. You just need to make it a habit, and you will begin to see results.

The equipment provides variety, but is not a necessity to create good exercise habits. Your own body can provide all of the equipment you need. You can learn those skills from a fitness trainer or for free, via videos from reputable sources, on the Internet.

Working with a qualified trainer is the safest and most effective way to learn new exercises. However, if affordability is a factor, then use the free means at your disposal.

Your Battle Plan

1) What types of exercise do you currently do?

2) What exercises or sports do you wish you could do now?

3) What sort of adaptations or modifications would be needed for you to participate in that sport?

4) Are you willing to at least try?

7. Rock Steady Boxing

Rock Steady Boxing (RSB) is a non-profit organization whose exercise program is designed specifically to benefit those of us diagnosed with Parkinson's disease. It is the product of one man seeking a way to battle his own diagnosis a couple of decades ago. I am blessed to know him and the former world champion women's boxer who trained with him. Together, they developed this program which is now available at over 900 locations worldwide. I am fortunate to count them among my friends.

RSB will work you harder than you may have ever worked in your entire life. It does not matter if you are physically fit, or use a cane, a walker, a wheelchair, have a bad knee, a bad hip, or suffer from other physical ailments. These specially-trained coaches can adapt and modify their program to fit your abilities.

Next, they will inspire and challenge you to amaze yourself with what you can achieve. I have witnessed people discovering that they are able to do things they didn't think possible.

The first time you witness or attend a class, it may seem overwhelming. When you encounter an eighty-year-old grandma who can outrun and outjump you, that's motivation. There have been cases of people leaving the gym and forgetting to take their walkers with them.

I've witnessed members arrive at this program and transform within the first few months. They become stronger, more agile, more confident, more flexible. I love seeing someone who hasn't run in forty years and watch them progress from walking, to running, to sprinting over time. They grow from performing the most basic forms of exercises into much more challenging and complex versions. The bravery in taking that first step and allowing yourself to attempt something that seems so out of character is a massive victory.

I've learned to jump rope in my sixties. I'm not ready for Double Dutch or anything, but I can jump rope. Heck, just recently, I watched two older women who were jumping together, using one standard jump rope. Afterward, they proceeded over to the hula hoops and did that for awhile. Until you have experienced this program, it is hard to even imagine.

It was great to be a spectator as these two women were reliving childhood memories by doing things that most people their age view as impossible or too dangerous to attempt.

No matter what your ability, there is an exercise routine for you. In addition to the grueling workouts, they offer modified versions. Routines can be done in a straight-back chair. And they have specialized routines for wheelchair users. If you have a chronic injury or limitation, the coaches are ready to show you adaptations. Members in wheelchairs punch heavy bags and speed bags. Others with walkers perform core-strengthening exercises on the gym floor. Miracles happen within those gym walls. That's how I see it. If you cannot attend class in person, for whatever reason, there are Internet options for participating.

A great side benefit of the RSB program is the friendships you make. We work very hard in our workouts, and we share conversation and laughter. You genuinely will become like family with some of your fellow boxers. PwPD have a unique understanding of each other. Not only do we exercise and sweat together, we go out to eat and attend social and athletic events. Our group has had picnics, cycling events, yoga in the park, holiday parties, golf outings, an organized motorcycle ride, and a political rally at the state capitol for PD awareness. We've held movie nights and ventured out to the ballet and roller derby.

Rock Steady is not the only exercise program available. It just happens to be one of the biggest and the one with which I am most familiar. I believe there are other boxing-based workouts. There are also PD dancing programs, Tai Chi, and swimming classes.

Opportunities abound to keep living well. Explore which programs are available in your own area, either in person or via the Internet. Don't be intimidated to go try them out. Everyone participating in these programs is facing the same disease as you. Join them. Be proactive, and fight for your quality of life.

Your Battle Plan

1) What exercise options for Parkinson's are available where you live?

2) What about the Internet options?

3) Have you checked out Parkinson's exercise workouts on Internet videos?

8. Doreen's Story

Receiving information about your health, especially if it is a difficult disease without a cure, is a shock to *hear* let alone *accept*. I was numb and disheartened, feeling the sense of path was already picked for me, with little options.

I had just retired about six months earlier and got COVID within one week, during the time so many were dying without any vaccines or meds to assist. Then, six months later, I was diagnosed with Parkinson's. What a start for retirement. But that is exactly what it was, a *start*, not a *finish*.

I had seven symptoms that then dwindled down to one! Why? Because I found steps to take that not only helped the physical symptoms but helped me to start taking action and writing the story myself versus the experience being predetermined and jammed down my psyche and burdening my heart.

I immediately joined Rock Steady Boxing. Yes, the physical action helped remove some symptoms, but it was the connection with community that also made the difference. I believe in the concept of "energy follows thought." I took steps to join others in using the practice but also living the message—you can *rock* this! I not only found a variety of health steps to take, but I learned about the steps my heart and mind can take to be vulnerable and open at the same time. Processing *all* feelings, not shutting down any of them, and knowing I was not alone. Everyone's journey is unique. Take steps that work for *you*. Remember there are actions that make a difference, and they start with you.

— Doreen, 68 years old

9. Attitude

Your attitude toward your new reality is something that will definitely impact your success or lack thereof. No matter how perfectly you do things, you will have challenging days. I refer to those as my "off" days. I must make room for them in my life. They are part of the PD experience.

An off day is typically one where I am completely exhausted. I do not necessarily feel sick or poorly, I just have zero energy in the tank. It is a sensation where I could literally lie motionless for the entire day, with nothing on my mind, and be perfectly content. I now plan for such days during my travels or during my normal life routine. I must remain aware that sometimes I need to take it easy for a day and allow my energy to return. This is okay. It is not a reason for frustration. The key is to not allow it to become a habit.

I view Parkinson's disease as an adversary. One of its primary objectives is to convince me to be as sedentary as possible. The less active I am, physically and mentally, the more opportunity the disease has to progress and gain an advantage over me. PD is relentless in its pursuit of convincing me to stop living. I can never give in to the temptation for any extended period of time. Yes, I take a day off, but I do not permit myself to remain that way for very long. I've witnessed this to be the quickest road to failure when battling this disease. Inactivity cannot be permitted to become the norm.

Parkinson's will also throw various symptoms at you which can be debilitating. When one strikes, seek treatment relentlessly. Do not accept the problem and allow it to dictate your life, be proactive in preventing your symptoms from slowing you down and gaining more control.

For the nerve pain I mentioned earlier, I tried numerous options, not all were helpful. However, I didn't consider any of the treatments to be failures. Instead, I viewed them as learning experiences. If you do not attempt a solution, then it will never succeed. *That* is the definition of failure. If you give a treatment a complete effort, and it is unsuccessful, you did not fail. You gained knowledge. Taking this approach, I discovered solutions which keep me functioning when these issues occur.

It doesn't matter if you need to see ten different doctors, try three different medications, or utilize various therapies, keep going until you have a satisfactory answer.

PD inflicts a variety of symptoms. You are not likely to experience them all. You will deal with your own custom set of challenges. Here are some of the more common symptoms, but certainly not a complete listing: hand tremors, arm tremors, leg tremors, body (torso) tremors, tongue tremors, eye tremors, muscle stiffness, balance issues, difficulty standing, difficulty walking, involuntary body movements, muscle rigidity, lack of coordination, rhythmic muscle contractions, muscle freezing, slowed movements, restless sleep, nightmares, vivid dreams, sleep disturbances such as flailing of arms and legs, fatigue, dizziness, amnesia, confusion, hoarseness, weak vocal volume, voice box spasms, anxiety, apathy, lost or distorted sense of smell, incontinence, blank stare, difficulty swallowing, falling, depression, neck tightness, small handwriting, and drooling. While that list may be overwhelming or downright scary, you can manage or minimize many of these with a good plan and a strong will.

Your outlook on your condition can also be positively impacted by getting involved in the Parkinson's community in your area. Exercise groups, support groups, social groups, and outreach organizations can all be ways to connect with other

PwPD. Surrounding yourself with people who ask the same questions and face the same obstacles is a great bonding experience. I make many friends this way. We share almost a familial bond and socialize together. We go to restaurants, have picnics, do seminars, and attend charitable events. We laugh together often, cry together on occasion, and love one another in a positive way. There is an understanding that exists with others battling this disease.

I cannot stress enough the fact that your life continues after diagnosis. Time doesn't stop. Neither should you. Focus on making today the very best day that it can be. Make the most of it, and fully live in the present. Before you know it, you will string together a whole bunch of great todays. That's when you rediscover joy, and Parkinson's has to take a backseat to the rest of the important things in your life.

Your Battle Plan

1) How's your attitude?

2) Which symptoms are challenging you?

3) Do you find it hard to get motivated?

4) Would you benefit from a helper encouraging you and keeping you motivated?

10. Diet

Most of us love to eat. It is more than just essential, it is enjoyment and entertainment. The myriad of food choices available to us is much greater than our ancestors' choices. I love the diversity and variety of the selections in our restaurants and grocery stores.

In my little neighborhood, there are typical American grocers, a few Mexican markets, some Asian markets, Indian markets, an Amish bakery, and a Middle Eastern grocery store. Those are all within a couple of miles, and that is most likely an incomplete list. I often see foods I do not recognize in these places. Vegetables and fruits from certain regions of the world are completely foreign to me. It depends upon your own level of culinary adventurousness as to how many of these items you might try.

Let me share one of my recent discoveries. I've always liked radishes, but I've learned that a few cultures eat pickled radishes. I never imagined such a thing, but it is great for my taste buds.

Another recent discovery is the Brookie. That's a brownie topped with a cookie and baked together.

Although, I won't be eating them very often or else I will gain an extra hundred pounds!

Enough with the swooning about foods, let's discuss the importance of choosing what you eat with Parkinson's disease. Your individual journey will dictate how you adjust your diet.

Many PD patients lose a great deal of weight, others do not. Some can handle things such as caffeine just fine, while others will notice their tremors increase. That's me. Caffeine causes me to tremor significantly more. Too much sugar can also have a similar impact on some of us.

Many foods we purchase are highly processed and contain additives and preservatives. These chemicals can be triggers. There is no way to know ahead of time which foods or chemicals will affect you. It is imperative that you are aware and take note of how different foods alter how you are feeling.

What I have discovered for myself is that a "clean diet" works best. What do I mean by a clean diet? It means that I strive to eat foods in their most natural forms. I try to consume raw fruits, raw vegetables, and meats without added flavors, colors, or preservatives. I avoid added sugars, eat more whole grains, nuts, and seeds, and stay away from foods that are processed for convenience. That being said, I can eat anything once in awhile as a treat, but even then, I make improved choices in my selections.

As an example, I absolutely love ice cream. That's not a health food, but I can choose a brand that has a listing of ingredients I recognize. If I cannot pronounce it, I probably shouldn't eat it. That's how I read food labels.

Currently, next to me is a bag of tortilla chips. The ingredients are: corn flour, water, vegetable oil, and sea salt. That's all. I recognize all of those ingredients, so that is something I will eat.

For dinner this evening, I will make a salad. I am planning to use romaine lettuce, radishes, cucumbers, turnips, onions, swiss cheese, pistachio nuts, almonds, an avocado, and a vinegar dressing. I will feel very satisfied by that. The nuts add a richness and texture to the salad that makes it complete. Later, I will eat a small piece of dark chocolate and maybe some olives. I've decided that snacks with a bolder flavor profile satisfy me more than the milder ones.

Again, you need to do you, but what you eat will impact how you feel and whether your PD symptoms lessen or worsen. In my world, I experience less pain, less tremoring, and less apathy, if I am vigilant about my diet. One last thing I do is drink water 95% of the time. Occasionally, I will sip on a cup of hot tea or some juice, but water is my beverage of choice.

You need to continue to be actively involved in meal preparation at home. It may require adjustments, and you might be more messy about it, but retaining those skills for as long as possible will do you a world of good.

I try to be mindful, but I may nick a finger more frequently. Sometimes, I forget to turn off a faucet or leave the fridge door open. Oh well, all I can do is laugh about it and keep moving. I also use the automatic dishwasher less. Handwashing the dishes is a good functional activity for my finer motor skills.

Your Battle Plan

1) How often do you check food labels?

2) Can you make a list of healthy foods that you enjoy?

3) What is your least healthy treat?

4) How can you make healthier versions of your treats?

5) Which foods or drinks cause your PD symptoms to be worse?

11. Medications

Parkinson's medications are a daily fact of life for the majority of PD patients. It is a balancing act of finding the correct drugs and dosages for controlling an ever-changing disease. It is crucial to maintain regular communications with your doctor(s) and your pharmacist. Utilize their expertise and knowledge. Anything from changes in your symptoms to various drug side effects can be addressed and improved, if you keep communications open. Expect your circumstances to be fluid. That's not a cause for alarm. Your personal situation may worsen or improve as time goes on, depending upon other factors in your life.

Be open to all possibilities, until you determine what works best for you. You may need to try different drugs, or you may be a candidate for other treatments.

Let me share an encouraging tidbit. I am friends with one individual who improved so much through exercise that she was able to stop taking PD medications last summer. The reason I share this is to reassure you that not all changes ahead will necessarily be negative.

One popular treatment that select PD patients qualify for is a Deep Brain Stimulation implant. The device is surgically placed into your brain and is intended to control tremors by delivering a mild electrical current into targeted areas of the brain. This helps neurons to communicate better with one another. The implant is not a good option for everyone, but I do know a few people who have had exceptional results. It is not a decision to be made lightly. There are complications to consider, and this option will only be beneficial for patients with certain types of Parkinson's symptoms. It is a discussion to have with your doctor, especially if you are not well-controlled with medications.

I am not discussing specific medications because I am not qualified to do so. That is a conversation for you to have with your own specialist. I can, however, tell you my personal situation. I am currently on zero Parkinson's drugs. The neurologist who diagnosed me was of the belief that if you can control your symptoms in other ways, then do so as long as possible before beginning PD meds. I have been extremely fortunate to be able to manage well with diet, exercise, and great medical therapies to this point. When the time comes that I need the drugs, that is perfectly fine with me. But, for now, I am doing well about eight and a half years in by doing the things I do.

Most of my PD friends do take varying amounts of the drugs. It all depends upon an individual's disease progression. Yes, those off days sometimes feel like I might need a pill, but my PD friends have those days too. That's the Parkinson's apathy, the feeling that you have zero energy to do anything. I do take a couple of regular medications—a blood pressure pill and a cholesterol pill. So, I am not against taking drugs. I also take vitamin E and vitamin D daily. Those are indeed due to probable Parkinson's side effects. I just don't require a true PD drug yet.

These are very individualized topics to cover with your healthcare team. You must decide what is working the best, and be proactive in your own care. Advocate for yourself for options and solutions to suit your own circumstances.

Your Battle Plan

1) Are you on any specific Parkinson's drugs?

2) How is your medication working?

3) Have you discussed any concerns with your doctor or pharmacist?

4) Which side effects should you discuss with your medical team at your next visit?

12. Young-Onset Parkinson's Disease (YOPD)

Those of us who were diagnosed at a younger age, I'd call it before age sixty, face some different circumstances than our older counterparts. We will be living with PD for decades to come. Many of us still work or have children at home. We may face increased responsibilities and a less settled existence. We might have other medical issues.

Being younger, we are more likely to suffer from the "Why me?" syndrome. It hardly seems fair to have to deal with such a serious condition at a young age. Denial, depression, and anger are common reactions. We might try to hide our condition. Younger people are more apt to isolate themselves because we're embarrassed, scared, or insecure. There might be a tendency to avoid public settings, so we do not need to constantly explain.

Let's be real, most people have seen a shaky old person and assume they have PD or a similar ailment.

When we see a shaky younger individual, we jump to the conclusion that they must be drunk or high. Parkinson's doesn't come to mind.

There are advantages to being younger with PD. We are less likely to fall and less likely to injure ourselves when we do fall. Our bones are stronger. We tend to be more flexible than our older counterparts. Our progression might be slower, and our options for maintaining functionality are frequently more varied. Typically, we are not facing as many other medical conditions simultaneously.

Getting involved in the Parkinson's community was a fabulous decision for me. First, I met people who were going strong after decades of proper self-care. They are living examples of how to succeed with this disease. The wealth of knowledge they possess and share is invaluable. Their positive attitudes and winning spirits demonstrate they are genuinely living happy lives.

The second benefit of being involved in the Parkinson's community is that I have met people my age or younger than me. We have become each other's role models. Additionally, we have become the closest of friends. There are a few I would even call family. We share experiences and tackle downright crazy adventures together. We make memories, great memories. Gaining new friends from getting involved in exercise programs, support groups, social activities, focused events, social media, and the Internet is a gift. Discovering others who know and understand your situation provides a nurturing and supportive environment.

As a YOPD person, I encourage you to not give up on your favorite activities. Adaptations can be made for most of them. I mentioned previously that I switched to a recumbent three-wheel bike. This enables me to keep making the long cycling rides I enjoy.

After a long day, I take a soaking bath. It refreshes me. My balance is good these days, but occasionally I experience a wobbly day. To be proactive, I installed a grab bar for safety. Better to have it and not need it than to need it and not have it.

When engaged in strenuous activities, I take more frequent breaks. No matter what the task or adventure, I try not to be foolish.

I owned a small business for many years where I scaled house roofs a couple of times a week. I don't do that anymore. I send someone else up there if I need work done. Most of the time, my balance is okay. But it only takes a split second for my balance to go haywire, and I would be in trouble. Better safe than sorry.

Here is an odd factoid I've learned with YOPD. If you are stopped by police for anything, inform them you have Parkinson's disease. It can prevent misunderstandings where they think you are under the influence of an illegal substance or drunk. That information may seem like it's out in left field, but it is something to keep in mind.

With YOPD, you can certainly have concerns with your career. Most employers will attempt to accommodate your disability, within reason. However, depending on your individual circumstances, you may need to change careers or retire earlier than expected. There is no shame in making changes to take care of yourself and your family. We all face unexpected changes from time to time.

If you have children, be open and honest with them about having YOPD. They may not express it, but they are going to worry about you. Let them know that you are going to be okay and that you aren't going to disappear. Be involved and engage with them. Be open when you experience symptoms, but do not cause them unnecessary stress. They don't deserve the burden. They deserve your continued attention, positivity, and your love. Your family didn't ask for this any more than you did, so it is your responsibility to maintain your relationships and demonstrate that you are fine. Include them in your exercise routines. Do activities together regularly. Make lots of new memories and ensure your days are meaningful. You will never regret choosing to create positive experiences with your family.

My final suggestion for you with YOPD concerns doctors' visits. You may not be accustomed to visiting doctors and therapists regularly. Get over that. Go and get all of the support and treatments you need. Take your medications. Go for check-ups and follow-ups. Don't try to just tough it out. That attitude will be detrimental in the long run. Your medical care team is part of your new reality, and they are there to help you maintain a high quality of life. Utilize their expertise.

Your Battle Plan

1) What are your biggest challenges?

2) What can you do today to improve that situation?

3) How can you help your family to adjust to this new reality?

13. Longevity

One of the first questions you want answered when you are diagnosed is, "How long do I have left to live?" Naturally, we cannot help but wonder if this is going to kill us. While Parkinson's disease itself won't kill you, it could be a contributing factor. This longevity question is a bit more complex than it may appear on the surface. Are you in rather early stages, or are your symptoms more advanced? What other health issues do you have already? How old are you?

Hey, let's face it, if you are diagnosed as being in the early stages of PD at the age of ninety-five, it is not likely to be much of a factor in your lifetime. However, if you are forty years old, then you need to figure out how to have a good and productive life for many decades to come. Is that possible? Absolutely!

I personally know people diagnosed decades ago who are doing well, even thirty or forty years later. They are typically the ones who kept on living and even took on additional challenges to improve their health after diagnosis. I know that I am healthier now than I was at the time of my diagnosis eight and a half years ago.

Back then, I would have been exhausted quickly from attempting to run. I would have been limited in the numbers of push-ups and sit-ups. Balancing on one foot and flexibility exercises would have been challenging. Now, I am several years into my PD journey and truthfully more fit than most average people half my age! I am not saying this to brag. I am saying this because I am truly shocked. I could have never imagined feeling this good in my sixties. It was a gradual progression, and I have Parkinson's to thank for that. It was my motivation to keep pushing forward.

I hope that my story somehow helps to motivate you to surprise yourself as well. I truly believe we are often far more capable than we give ourselves credit for. I know PD can do nasty things. This is why we need to work hard to reduce its effect on our daily lives.

I recall a conversation between two coaches, at my local Rock Steady Boxing gym. The coaches, who worked with PwPD for over a decade, discussed the passing of one of our members from cancer. He was in his seventies and had been an active member of our PD community. The two coaches considered the fact that in all of their years working with PwPD, they couldn't remember one case of someone whose cause of death was PD. The causes were usually heart disease, stroke, cancer, pneumonia, all the same normal stuff that eventually claims everyone else.

The gym is a close family. We keep in touch, even after a member can no longer attend in-person sessions due to health concerns. To me, this was quite a profound revelation coming from coaches who have literally known thousands of people with this disease.

Does this mean that nobody dies from significant Parkinson's complications? Of course not. There are some serious situations that can arise, due to aspiration or a bad fall, where PD would be a major factor. Parkinson's dementia and hallucinations can be considered as causes that lead to someone's passing. But, for the people who have chosen to be proactive, to keep moving, to keep exercising, the outcomes are typically better.

I have taken part in a couple of major university research studies analyzing the benefits of an active lifestyle for people with Parkinson's disease. They tracked my abilities over a period of time to see how much my physical and mental functions improved with increased exercise. It is proving to be a big leap forward in managing this disease.

Sorry, I tend to veer off-topic at times. Back to longevity, if you do an Internet search of life expectancy with PD, it will give you an answer of perhaps ten to twenty years. But, that answer is too simplistic and hardly fair. Of course, a ninety-five-year-old isn't expecting another twenty years, and the forty-year-old is hoping for far more. Those numbers also fail to consider other health risk factors or the actual cause of death. When you dig deeper into the numbers, many people are diagnosed with Parkinson's at an advanced age.

My own research and observations have resulted in my viewing this disease as having a less significant negative impact on longevity. As long as you remain proactive in your care and do the proper things to maintain or improve your healthy lifestyle, your quality of life will be better than if you sit on the couch and do nothing.

Your Battle Plan

1) Are you doing all that you can to maintain or improve your quality of life?

2) What things can you improve?

3) Who can help you to reach your longevity goals?

PART II
COMMON SYMPTOMS

I am devoting this section of the book to specific symptoms that are common but perhaps less addressed in your journey. We all know about the tremors. That's the most identifiable symptom. However, we face a potpourri of other maladies that can also impact our daily lives.

14. Short-Term Memory

Someone recently asked me where I watched last year's Super Bowl and who was there. I told them that I had no idea, no clue. This made me think about last Fourth of July. Where was I? Again, no idea. My last birthday, where did I go? What did I do? I struggled with the questions. Eventually, I recalled what I did on my exact birthday. I went to a concert I'd been eager to attend. But, I cannot remember when or where we had my family birthday celebration. I know it would have been on a different day, due to me attending the concert, but as for other details, I have none.

If you asked me what I did yesterday, I could give you a good summary. But, if you asked about the day before, or last week, I most likely wouldn't have an answer.

Certain memories may be triggered, due to regularity. However, details of other events escape me. Six days ago, I went to boxing class. Why do I know this? Well, because 99% of the time, I go to boxing that day every week. I recall there were eighteen people in the class that day. What was the workout? I do not remember.

A few weeks ago, I received an advertisement via e-mail from a hardware chain. One of the sale items in particular caught my attention as something I could use. It was a set of handy adapters to use with socket wrenches. This would be an inexpensive and useful purchase for projects I do around the house. So, I printed out the special coupon and drove, out of my way, to the store to obtain these adapters. I was all happy about it.

A couple of days later, I carried my adapter set to the basement to hang on the pegboard in my workshop. Imagine my surprise when I found an identical set of adapters hanging, in an unopened package, on the pegboard in my workshop. Apparently, I bought them on a previous trip to the same store in the past.

Although memory issues can come with aging or with other conditions, it is more common with Parkinson's disease.

My long-term memory appears to be unaffected. I remember many specific details of events, places, smells, and sensations from fifty years ago. Last week, last month, or five years ago present more of a problem.

I could focus on the memory loss in a negative way and get depressed. Instead, I choose not to dwell on it. On the lighter side, I get to watch television shows or movies for the first time multiple times over. It's like always having new entertainment.

In an attempt to preserve more recent events, I've decided to keep a daily journal. That way, I can refer back to it to recall certain events and experiences. Journaling provides a detailed reference guide to my daily life that has proven quite beneficial. I highly recommend it.

Your Battle Plan

1) How is your short-term memory?

2) How is your long-term memory?

3) Would you benefit from keeping a memory journal?

15. Brain Fog

Brain fog is a term you will hear regularly among Parkinson's patients. It is an appropriate term to describe the lack of clarity or control we will sometimes experience. It reminds me of how an old car behaved when it had gotten some bad gas. The engine would sputter and the car might lurch and shake. Things would just go awry. It still ran, but not very smoothly.

In my opinion, brain fog actually encompasses several different anomalies. The most prominent feature is a lack of clarity. You just don't feel with it or on top of your game. Mental slowness would be an alternate way to describe this sensation. You aren't as alert or mentally nimble as usual. That can be accompanied by slower movements as well. The slowed movements are frequently associated with the fact that the signals aren't moving from your brain to your muscles in a timely manner. Those signals sputter and cause havoc.

I will tell my hand to do something, and it won't cooperate because the message received is all jumbled and confused. My poor hand tries its best, but it is being fed bad data. I use my hand as an example, but this can occur in multiple areas of your body—feet, legs, arms, tongue, head, neck, and torso. If there are muscles present, you may experience communication problems.

A pure lack of mental focus is a symptom of brain fog. Staying on task can be a major challenge. I believe this is why learning new things is so important. It requires you to remain focused on the task at hand. You may struggle with reading an owner's manual or following a recipe because you cannot keep your mind on task. You may be taking pills and have difficulty remembering which ones you just swallowed because you weren't paying attention. This is a good advertisement for one of those medication organizers.

We often hear about the blank, emotionless facial expressions of someone with Parkinson's. A portion of this can be attributed to brain fog. I cannot speak for everyone, but I can literally be thinking of absolutely nothing at times. I tell my friends it's my "nothing box." Twenty years ago, I wouldn't have believed that was even possible. Now, it is a most relaxing place. It is quite peaceful in there.

Brain fog can contribute to impulsive and destructive behaviors as well. When you are enjoying an activity such as gambling, your lack of focus may cloud your normally good judgement regarding when to quit.

Be certain to discuss brain fog with your loved ones. It can help them understand when you aren't responding or behaving in a manner that they recognize. Make sure they comprehend that it is not because you do not care or lack interest. It is the Parkinson's. Of course, you have a responsibility to fight this symptom daily as well. Good lifestyle choices and appropriate medication can ease these episodes. Effort and understanding from everyone in your personal realm can go a long way toward minimizing the negative effects.

Your Battle Plan

1) Have you experienced moments of brain fog or confusion?

2) Do you have difficulty concentrating or staying on task?

3) Have you discussed your brain fog with loved ones and your doctors?

16. Apathy

The "apathy monster" is definitely real with Parkinson's disease. The strong urge to do absolutely nothing and live as a sloth can be overwhelming at times. Unfortunately, that is the absolute worst thing a PwPD can do. The lethargy will overtake you rapidly if you sit or lie around all day. You will feel you do not have the energy nor the desire to move a muscle voluntarily. The disease will attempt to convince you that nothing matters and that you are too exhausted to care.

Remember—that is the disease talking. Do not listen! Get your butt moving. Get your brain moving. Get busy. Keep living. There will be plenty of time to lie around and do nothing once you are dead.

Until then, make the most of every single moment. You must focus on moving every day. Go for a walk. Do the laundry. Work on a jigsaw puzzle. Do arm curls with soup cans. If you are physically able, then go for a run, jump rope, make a special dinner, or go volunteer at a charity that has meaning to you. Do anything you can to engage in life. Do it, and do it regularly.

As previously mentioned, it's healthy to take a day off occasionally. Just ensure you do not allow this behavior to become a habit or the norm. After a rest day, you must get busy again.

Personally, I found that the first step is the hardest. Once I begin one task, I flow right into the next one and the next. Before I know it, my day is humming along. Sure, I take more frequent breaks than I once did. They are necessary. Just always be aware that they are also opportunities for the apathy monster to take over again.

My suggestion is at the beginning of your break, tell yourself how long this break will last and stick to it. Keep yourself accountable. Set an alarm, preferably one you have to get up and walk over to in order to turn off. Now, you're up. And once you're up, you're up. That's half the battle. Now, you can tackle a task or do something fun. It's up to you. Either way, you will feel better about yourself both mentally and physically.

Time will not stand still and wait for you. Strive to live each day fully. Make the most of these days, and do not give up.

Your Battle Plan

1) How are you battling apathy?

2) What prevents you from keeping busy?

3) What are you doing today to keep your mind and body active?

17. That Blank Face

I have read that approximately 40% of Parkinson's sufferers will have the blank, emotionless face. That's a fairly large number. I am of the belief that we also tend to express or process less emotion. It doesn't mean we are unfeeling or uncaring. Our feelings can get hurt, and unfortunately, we are able to hurt others. Some of the tools usually utilized for our emotional health are lacking. PwPD must work on being more animated, more outgoing, and more outwardly enthusiastic. That will involve conveying to our family and friends when we are enjoying ourselves or when they are appreciated. Making a more conscious effort to be expressive is required. Without this, others may get the wrong impressions that they are not important to us or that we are not enjoying time with them.

Concentrating on expression is especially crucial in interactions with your spouse, significant other, and your children. You may inadvertently be giving off negative vibes that suggest that you do not care or that they are unimportant to you. This could unintentionally cause serious harm to your relationship.

The apathy monster can exacerbate the situation and you may think that you don't care. You may feel as if it doesn't matter if this person disappears from your life or that nothing really matters. And while relationships fail every day, make certain that your Parkinson's is not the primary reason for your bad situation. You don't want to realize a week or a month too late that you destroyed or severely damaged your relationship with a loved one. They can't be expected to determine whether it is you or the disease talking. Do your best not to cause unnecessary harm for the wrong reasons.

Your Battle Plan

1) Who is most important to you?

2) Have you told them today?

3) Are you working on being more expressive?

4) Are you communicating your appreciation?

18. Mobility

Episodes of mobility problems can be very frustrating. Many people shuffle, often they fall, sometimes they even freeze. All of these can be demoralizing and even dangerous. Safeguarding against the more serious outcomes, while also striving to maintain your personal dignity and independence, is crucial.

Parkinson's exercise programs are incredibly effective in helping you retain or improve mobility. I observe people every week who are running, jumping, rolling, and falling on purpose. We actually practice falling, in order to learn how to do so without injuring ourselves. We practice how to stand and move with a more solid base or foundation, to maintain balance and prevent falls in the first place.

When we do fall, the first reaction is to ensure we are okay, uninjured. Next, if possible, we stand back up on our own. Exercising and practicing standing techniques help us to be able to do this when needed. That being said, if you *do* require assistance, do not refuse help or get angry with those offering assistance. Be grateful to your helper for lending a hand.

I am reminded of a time when I attended a Parkinson's support group meeting. We sat around a table. One fellow was rejoining our group when he suddenly fell to the floor. Nobody panicked. We asked if he was okay. He responded in the affirmative. Then, he returned to his feet, on his own, without any fuss. Outsiders may view that as cruel, but everyone at the table had PD. We all understood it was necessary for him to have the opportunity to stand on his own. Had he needed assistance, we would have provided it. My point is that just because we have PD, it doesn't necessarily mean we are helpless.

That being said, if you require a cane, a walker, or a wheelchair, please use it! There are valid reasons for these devices. They are meant to improve quality of life. My Parkinson's exercise gym has many members who utilize such things. There is no shame. They are equal members of our community.

While talking mobility, the next concern is freezing. I am fortunate not to have this affliction, but I know several PwPD who do. Freezing is not a well understood phenomenon by researchers. It often occurs in a tight space or a doorway, although, it can happen anywhere. People with freezing often describe it as feeling as if their feet are stuck to the floor. They cannot move them.

I remember one particular circumstance where a gentleman froze right in the middle of a busy doorway entering a conference room. He was having difficulty getting unstuck. We patiently waited for a few moments until he was able to get moving again. Knowledge and understanding in that circumstance were key. Fortunately, there are medications and physical therapies which can minimize these episodes. There are also specific tactics that are taught and employed at the moment of freezing to aid the sufferer in getting unstuck.

Be forward-thinking with respect to your home. Make decisions with your circumstances in mind. You may not want a home with stairs in a few years, or you can look into an electric mobility lift to safely take you up and down your stairs. You may want that next bathroom renovation to include grab bars near the toilet and shower, and possibly make the shower wheelchair accessible. Although these things might never be an issue for you, keep the potential eventualities in mind, when making significant future plans.

Your Battle Plan

1) What mobility issues are you facing?

2) Which things do you need to address for your own safety?

3) Would you benefit from utilizing medical devices?

4) Do you need to add grab bars in the bathroom?

5) Would you benefit from a mobility chair for a stairway?

19. Doug's Story

First, I'd like to thank Lynn for giving me the opportunity to present a synopsis of my story in this book. I start my small section with a question. Is Parkinson's a curse or a gift? In my opinion, it's been both, but mostly the latter. Let me explain.

In the fall of 2013, I was diagnosed with Young-onset Parkinson's disease (YOPD), at the ripe old age of forty-three. I could've been shocked by the diagnosis, but I was relieved, having imagined many worse possibilities. The biggest challenge I have faced with Parkinson's has been mobility. When I'm on medication and at my peak, I can run as fast as I want to, maybe even trying to catch up to the wind. When I'm off medication, I think grains of sand blowing in a breeze move faster than I can.

In 2016, I joined Rock Steady Boxing, at one of the local affiliates where I was living at the time. It was a game changer! The coach of the local affiliate pushed me and further cemented my love for intense exercise, as the way to therapeutically reinvigorate my body.

Rock Steady Boxing is not a cure, but rather a

means to slow disease progression. The constant battle of maintaining the normal existence of mobility has been the curse part of the disease for me, but the intense exercise turned Parkinson's into some of the greatest gifts I've ever had so far.

Fast forward about nine years in my life. I've moved to a new location with my family. I joined the Rock Steady Boxing home gym. That was scary and exciting at the same time. Scary, because the home gym's reputation was steeped in legend, and many coaches were part of folklore. Seriously though, I love it. As I had done in the affiliate, I pushed my body to the limits. I quickly earned the nickname, "Overachiever," all the while trying to push back the time dam Parkinson's invoked on my body and spirit. My spirit was strong, all due to the love of my family, supportive friends, and work colleagues.

The ninth year of my Parkinson's journey, so far, has been the most stressful time of my life. I was diagnosed with cancer and won't sugarcoat the fact that it absolutely terrified me. I mean nobody knows how they're gonna react when they truly face the aspect of potentially dying. Fortunately, the gift of intense exercise that I used to push my body through for all those years armored me for the cancer battle ahead.

I had six months of chemotherapy and then twenty radiation treatments to kill the cancer in my body. Fortunately, the physical shape I was in, which I considered banked in the assets column for the fight against cancer, kept me from getting sick and having a much worse situation. Radiation was the worst part of treatment because I lost my sense of taste. All food tasted like the same flavor of Play-Doh. Having such a drab sense of taste, I consumed as many empty calories as I could, just to keep my weight up. Imagine brushing your teeth at night and your eyes watering in pain because your mouth is on fire from the stimulation of the radiation.

Currently, I am in remission. Yay! I have had a few post-cancer health setbacks, but that's to be expected when you have that much therapy, mostly poor circulation and digestive issues. But those also impacted how I absorb and metabolize my medication. It slowed me down a bit. Some days, I am Mr. Overachiever and proud of it. Other days, I feel like the cartoon mouse, Slowpoke Rodriguez.

Overall, life with Parkinson's has given me more checkmarks in the "gift" column than in the "curse" column. What other gifts has Parkinson's given me? I have the courage to continually look at myself and figure out how to make a better version of me—mentoring in science, participating in PD clinical trials, playing old and learning new musical instruments, exploring new hobbies such as 3D printing, and performing car karaoke with my Parkinson's friends—that's one of my favorites.

— Doug, 53 years old

20. Destructive Behaviors

People with Parkinson's disease are more susceptible to self-destructive behaviors. These behaviors feed the pleasure centers of the brain. They are referred to as impulse control disorders. Examples include uncontrolled gambling, hypersexuality, compulsive shopping, kleptomania, and compulsive eating. You can make a bad decision in an instant that may have negative ramifications for a very long time.

I have a bit of a compulsion for shopping. Online shopping makes it easy. I can select an item and have it ordered in a matter of seconds. My personal saving grace is that my shopping habit is typically satisfied by inexpensive things I thought I couldn't do without at that very moment. Thank goodness for easy return policies! I am lucky that my issue is not one which causes any sort of damage to my life or my relationships.

I am aware of couples where the hypersexuality issue caused severe distress in their marriages. This compulsion can lead to unfortunate situations, causing a wedge between the spouses or even lead to infidelity.

If the problem is gambling, an individual's entire life savings can be decimated in short order and have nothing left to show for it. Winning fuels those pleasure centers in the brain. You win a jackpot, you feel great. However, people with impulse control issues may lose all of their winnings or end up chasing their losses attempting to find that brain chemical rush again.

Overeating causes additional health concerns, complicating your already challenging life. Aside from the obvious weight gain, you will feel more sluggish which will fuel increased apathy. The increased apathy will rationalize more overeating. And on it goes, becoming a vicious cycle.

Fortunately, support groups exist for each and every one of these compulsions. If you are feeling vulnerable, reach out and get the support you need before it complicates your life even further. Don't keep secrets. It's not your fault that you are facing this challenge. It only becomes your fault if you recognize the weakness and fail to seek solutions.

Your Battle Plan

1) Are you having any compulsive behaviors?

2) Are these behaviors causing problems in your relationships?

3) What do you need to do today to begin correcting these issues?

4) Who can help keep you accountable?

21. Vivid Dreams

The majority of people dream. I'm one of the lucky ones who remembers them. I've had fantastic, colorful dreams my whole life. I can even recall memorable ones from decades ago. The major difference with Parkinson's disease is that my dreams have become much more vivid, more elaborate, tremendously enjoyable, and entertaining.

I have been told by other PwPD that they experience vivid nightmares. I imagine that is quite unpleasant.

Fortunately, my dream experiences are 99% fun or fulfilling. I honestly look forward to them. They are a significant part of me, and I consider them my favorite PD symptom. One cautionary note concerning my dreams is they can be harmful to anyone nearby. I run, kick, and box actively while asleep. I once punched a nightstand so hard that my hand was sore for a week. I kicked a metal coffee table and ended up with a huge purple bruise to show for it. I'm lucky I didn't break my foot with that one. I added a small side rail to my bed because I kept rolling out. Any floor landing while sound asleep could prove dangerous. I've been fortunate to not be injured. Buying the bed rail wasn't very good for my ego, but it did reduce the risk of injury. My ego recovered just fine.

I live in a beautiful home in my dream-world. I can describe every room in great detail. I believe that it influenced my decision to buy my current house in the real world, as they have many similarities. I bought my home a year ago. I've been living in the dream-world version for much longer than that. In my dream-world, I also have an apartment in the city. I must be rich.

I am always working on projects or going on adventures during my nighttime saga. I also fly around, more like levitation I guess, but very cool. I compete in sporting events, solve crimes, and visit unusual places.

My adventures are random and unpredictable. The most perplexing part is when my dreams have surprising events or outcomes. How does my own mind surprise me? I haven't figured that out yet.

The absolute best part of my dreams is spending so much time with loved ones who are no longer alive. Their visits are wonderful, and we have long conversations. My father and I often work together in the workshop or share a favorite meal. Whether these visits are real or imagined, I don't know, and I don't care. All I know is that they have deep meaning and provide tremendous satisfaction to my heart and soul.

I hope that you have a PD dream-world that's as enjoyable as mine.

Your Battle Plan

1) Do you need to take safety precautions to protect you or others during sleep?

2) Have you considered journaling your dreams?

3) Who appears most often for a visit?

22. Other Common Challenges

A weak or raspy voice is quite common. Often, our voices become quieter and softer over time to the point to where we are difficult to understand during conversation. Additional voice issues include mumbling, slurring, and a monotone delivery. There are specific programs available that focus on vocal volume and quality. They teach and train you how to project your voice and enunciate more clearly.

I've noticed my own speaking voice weaken over time. I have not employed any specific therapies for it, but have been able to draw upon my past experiences with singing and public speaking. Those fields of study taught me to push from my abdomen when projecting my voice. This enables me to sound more robust.

Vocal programs will offer you targeted guidance for your own vocal weaknesses. The speech therapy program I am most acquainted with is called LSVT LOUD. They work with folks to boost their vocal abilities through various exercises and therapies. The organization also has a physical therapy and occupational therapy side. That's called LSVT BIG. They work with PwPD to increase the size of their movements to improve balance and stability.

Even if you do not exhibit much in the way of outward tremors with Parkinson's disease, you may struggle with fine motor skills. Those little, more subtle movements can be significantly impaired. Handwriting is certainly a fine motor skill. You might find yourself writing smaller and smaller. PwPD instinctively begin writing smaller as a control mechanism. It seems to be an intuitive adaptation to a motor skill problem. I am in that category. My handwriting was never good, but now it is noticeably smaller and still not good. It's hard to explain why my writing is this way. It just kinda happens. It goes back to those misfiring brain signals.

Fortunately, in today's world, handwriting is less essential, due to a world filled with keyboards and keypads. However, writing does still have a place, plus it is a good way to exercise those finer motor functions.

Do you remember when you were first learning to write that the teacher would give you papers with traceable letters and words to refine your skills? Well, I am here to tell you that those exercises work well with Parkinson's too! If your handwriting has become problematic, you may want to order some of those materials and relearn to write again. You can even take recess and go on the swings at the park in between lessons if you want. It's an opportunity to be a kid again!

Games can be helpful with finer motor skills. Remember playing the Operation game? Using tweezers to retrieve objects to avoid lighting up the red nose buzzer is great therapy. How about Pick-up Sticks? Those are two good games for practicing fine motor skills. You can tell people it's physical therapy. You don't need them to know you are also having fun.

Neuropathy can occur with many medical conditions including with PD. It's nerve damage that causes pain, numbness, weakness, or tingling anywhere in your body. The soles of my feet have significantly decreased sensation, almost as if I'm wearing a thick pair of socks. Also my hands tingle at times, along with nerve pain.

Some people respond well to medications for this, others benefit from acupuncture or massage to decrease severity. Neuropathy can be an ongoing, nagging, chronic problem with varying levels of severity. So, please keep your medical team informed and update your treatments as necessary.

The above mentioned conditions are only a few of the struggles you may face with Parkinson's disease. Many of these symptoms are not outwardly visible. So, it is essential for you to tell your doctor, your family, and your caregiver which symptoms you are experiencing. They cannot read your mind. Share with them, so they can understand and help you.

Now, back to keyboards for a moment. Those tremors and diminished fine motor skills will make your aim much worse when typing. Those darned fingers get lost during their journey to the appropriate keys. Of course, the smaller the keyboard, such as on a cell phone, the bigger the problem. I sometimes attempt to type a single sentence half a dozen times in order to get it right. It can be frustrating, but since I am stubborn, I keep going. You may discover that you repeat the exact same mistakes with your aim over and over again. That is a big pet peeve of mine. If I type the words, "interesting," "invest," or "intrigue," on my phone, I almost always type, "I nteresting," "I nvest," or "I ntrigue." Why, why, why? But, since I could have worse problems, I keep reminding myself that it is just a nuisance and not worth stressing over.

Your Battle Plan

1) What are your top challenges currently?

2) Are you actively pursuing therapies to address these issues?

3) Are you communicating your symptoms to your medical team? Your family?

23. This Is Too Much

If you are saying, "All of these ideas and various medical resources and exercise equipment and making the most of life, it's all wonderful, but I can't do all of that! I don't have the money or the time or the energy or the ability to do all of that!" Trust me, I do understand. I've struggled financially, emotionally, and physically at moments in my own life. I've barely survived extended periods of being overwhelmed, with no end in sight, and no good answers that I could find. I also realize that I am now this big ball of energy and positivity, and you may not be there. So, this chapter is for you.

I've stated previously, "Begin where you are." That philosophy is true in every aspect of life. The journey forward always begins with one step in the right direction. Parkinson's disease may cause an unanticipated change of direction, but do not allow the disease to become an impenetrable roadblock. Seek solutions. Most problems do indeed have a solution. It may not be your original plan, but find what works and run with it.

Depending on the demands of your job, continuing down your current path might not be a realistic possibility with PD. This can be a reason to feel down or defeated. But, what if you view it as an unexpected opportunity to pursue new goals, pursue new passions? Identify those new careers that you *can* do and that you would enjoy. Create a transition that works *for* you rather than *against* you.

You may have to apply for disability income. That's okay. That is why it is available to you. Use this benefit to move forward. Making this decision doesn't mean you need to go home and sit on the sofa.

Depending on your type of disability plan, you may be able to continue to work part-time or volunteer with an organization that is important to you. Fully explore these options, and find a path forward. Be the captain of your ship, and choose your course of action.

Please do not focus on what you cannot do. That serves you no good purpose. We all have things we cannot do. This isn't something unique to having Parkinson's. I can tell you with reasonable certainty that I will never play drums professionally again. It's just not in my future. The same might be true for your profession as a truck driver, a lawyer, or a teacher.

Your specific symptoms and afflictions may eliminate some possibilities, but there are other options available to you.

Similar limitations may occur in your recreational life. Circumstances with this disease are highly individualized. I know many PwPD who play golf regularly. I know some who still do cross-stitch and quilting. Whatever your hobbies, do not just quit, find modifications and workarounds to keep living your unique life.

I mentioned I now ride a three-wheel bike. I could lament the loss of my ability to safely ride a two-wheeler, but instead, I celebrate the fact that my new ride is much more comfortable on my back and my butt. It's actually an upgrade in many respects.

I have stressed that exercise is a key component of maintaining your quality of life. Honestly, this is a fact, not only for people with Parkinson's disease, but for every single human being. Yes, using fancy equipment, going to a gym, or having all of the right tools available would be great. However, you may not be able to afford any of those things right now. The most important habit you can form is to exercise every single day, with or without equipment.

Some of the greatest exercises you can do require nothing but your own body—push-ups, sit-ups, curls, burpees, planks, sit-to-stands, stretches, walking, running, or any other calisthenics you can imagine. Utilize things around the house, such as soup cans, milk jugs, basketballs, and baseballs. Be creative.

Need some fresh ideas? The Internet is filled with free workout videos. There are thousands specifically developed for Parkinson's people. We have a wealth of information available at our fingertips.

Yes, PD can cause dramatic changes to your life. Any change is difficult, ranging from minor nuisance to catastrophic disaster. PD hits you physically, mentally, and emotionally. You didn't want these changes. However, you must live with them.

Make the most of the opportunities available in your area. Keep living this new reality in a positive way every day, and before you know it, the new habits will become routine. It will require more effort at first, and you will need to make adjustments along the way. Just never ever stop. Keep moving forward. Keep fighting for what is yours. Keep creating your new life instead of just letting it happen to you. You can do this.

Your Battle Plan

1) Are you feeling overwhelmed? Who can you discuss this with?

2) What are two things you can do today to positively impact your PD?

3) Can you make a list of activities you enjoy that you are capable of doing?

PART III
THINGS TO CONSIDER

This section of the book proposes additional ideas and suggestions to consider as you navigate your present situation and the future ahead.

24. Steve's Story

A blessing disguised as a scourge. That is what Parkinson's is to me. I am stronger physically, mentally, and spiritually today as a result of the wake-up call by prostate cancer and Parkie twenty years ago.

First, I was blessed to have Parkinson's in Indianapolis, in 2007, the only place in the world at that time to experience the magic of Rock Steady Boxing. As my newfound fitness increased, many doors began to open. I found others who looked at the positive things that had happened in their lives because of their Parkinson's diagnosis, most of whom were more movement-challenged than I.

Following on the heels of my Rock Steady Boxing training, I began running competitively, in fourteen years, competing in over 130 events—from local races and 5Ks, to the Drake Relays in Iowa, and the Boston Marathon. I have climbed to 13,800 feet, hiking the Inca Trail with a group of Alzheimer's and Parkinson's advocates. I volunteer at the University of Indianapolis labs for physical therapy and occupational therapy students and serve as deacon at my church. The relationships and experiences throughout those years have enriched my life, as I have tried to give back as well.

I would not wish the ravages of Parkinson's on anyone. Sure, I would love to have a healthy brain and nervous system and prostate. But there can be life after diagnosis, if you focus on what you can do rather than what you can't do.

— Steve, 78 years old

25. Quality of Life

Earlier, we discussed the question of longevity. However, quality of life is probably our most pressing concern. We do not wish to merely exist. We desire to strive to enjoy and to make the most of our blessings. I cannot begin to speak to what brings you joy or what is important to you. All I can do is share my experiences.

In my younger years, I was a professional musician. I do not know that I could still perform concerts, at least not at a level I would consider satisfactory. I can, however, continue to learn, practice, and perform for my own entertainment. I conduct recording sessions where I redo sections to hide my mistakes. I also decided to learn to play a few new instruments, both because it is fun, and it is good exercise for my brain.

Music is like oxygen to me. It always has been, and will continue to be, an essential part of my life. Continuing these activities brings me great joy.

I love spending time with friends and family. I attend concerts and plays. I travel as much as possible. I tackle projects around the house. I'm currently working on a 1,000-piece jigsaw puzzle.

Whatever brings you joy, do it. Also, do not focus on what you cannot do. Focus on what you *can* do. I will repeat this sentiment often because it is *that* important. Identify the things you enjoy. Make any needed adaptations based upon your condition. Get busy living. You cannot change your age or the fact that you have been diagnosed with this disease. Concentrate on the things you can actually control. You can do this.

Your Battle Plan

1) What current activities bring you happiness?

2) What adaptations do you need to make now, if necessary, to live more fully?

3) Which additional activities can you add to benefit your body or mind?

26. My Personal Fitness Barometers

Due to the fact that the number of PwPD includes such a wide range in age and physical conditions, it is impossible for me to give many specific suggestions regarding exercise and fitness. However, I will share with you some of my own barometers for keeping tabs on how I am doing. Remember, I am a sixty-one-year-old man who has had PD for eight and a half years. I remain active as a part of my own battle plan.

At the beginning of this chapter of my life, I was an average guy in my early fifties. Now, I am a much more physically fit guy in my sixties. And let me tell you, that didn't happen overnight. It was a gradual progression through hard work, determination, dedication, and stubbornness. I don't resemble a bodybuilder. I don't have six-pack abs. But, I can run a mile, do fifty jumping jacks, and 100 sit-ups.

Let me use the sit-ups as an example. Ten years ago, I would have struggled at ten repetitions. I never would have guessed that 100 repetitions were possible in a million years. But, here I am today doing just that.

My personal fitness markers revolve around activities of daily living. Can I get down onto the floor and back up again without using my hands? That's a good barometer for me, to be able to do that easily. Now again, these are *my* personal markers. You may be better or worse than me.

Please do not try to get up off of the floor without using your hands, unless you can do so safely or have a spotter to catch you. You can't afford to injure yourself. For some people, just being able to get up from the floor without assistance can be a huge goal to achieve. For others, this may be an unrealistic expectation. You have got to do you. Begin where you are and improve from there.

Another good marker for me is a sit-to-stand exercise. How many times can I sit down and stand up from a chair in one minute? I am actually going to go do that right now, so I can give you my number. Don't go away, I will be right back.

I am now huffing and puffing, and my number of sit-to-stands in one minute was forty-three.

You may be able to crush that number or you may be at three. It does not matter. If you complete three today, can you increase to four tomorrow? That's how you make progress.

My next measure is the time it takes to run a mile. I run like a turtle, so my time is approximately eleven minutes.

If you can only walk ten feet today before you need to sit down, can you walk eleven tomorrow and twelve the next day? Any progress is progress.

Balance is a biggie for me. How long can I stand on one foot? Let me do that one really quick to get my numbers.

My right foot—one minute and forty-two seconds. My left foot—two minutes and three seconds.

You may need to stand on both feet or use a cane or a walker. Adjust to whatever fits your current situation. Put a chair in front of you or have someone there to assist you, if needed. Safety first!

Can I bend over and touch my toes? Nowadays, the answer is, "Yes." It used to be nearly impossible.

How long can I hold a ten-pound hand weight over my head? If ten pounds is not the right weight for you, choose a weight that makes you comfortable.

How long can I hold a plank position? How long can I hold a bridge position? These are a few of my favorite physical markers to measure how I am doing.

The overall message is that you can improve from where you are one day, one step, one movement at a time. You have that power.

Your Battle Plan

1) What physical markers are you ready to begin measuring?

2) What is a longer-term goal you would like to achieve?

3) Are you willing to begin today?

27. Social Life

You have Parkinson's disease. You have told your friends, family, and coworkers. Do you now just stay at home and not be seen in public? Will others treat you poorly? Will you be stared at, made fun of, excluded? Should you be insecure? The short answer is, "No," emphatically, "No!"

You may reach a point where you require a caregiver, especially if you are already older. This is a true statement for any person, not just individuals with Parkinson's.

Public activities can be daunting for some people with Parkinson's disease (PwPD). Going out to dinner may require that you bring your own weighted utensils. Going to a location where there is a lot of walking may require you to make use of a cane, a walker, or a wheelchair. Don't be ashamed. Just do it, and keep going. I know PwPD in their forties who use a cane or walker. And I know others, in their eighties, who can run for miles, so you may not face these issues. Either way, keep going.

You may find that being seated for too long at a play or concert feels uncomfortable. Take extra walks to stretch your muscles as needed.

I was in that type of situation last summer. I was on an overseas flight. Sitting in a stationary position for hours became overwhelming, so I trekked to the bathroom multiple times. I'm sure my fellow passengers thought I sure did pee a lot, but I was exercising my legs and stretching, using up my pent-up energy.

While on the subject of travel, you can and should be out exploring the world for as long as possible. I find that booking my itinerary lighter, and allowing an extra day here and there for rest, makes my trips much more enjoyable.

When planning your vacations, explain your specific needs and limitations to your traveling companions. While they might agree to alter activities to suit your condition, you can also allow them to understand that it is perfectly acceptable if they do activities without you.

Four years ago, I went to Disney World with my adult children. I accompanied them in the mornings, and we enjoyed various activities together. About midday, I returned to the hotel for a nap. The rest of the family kept going. Then, we resumed joint activities later in the day. It worked out great. Everyone was satisfied with the arrangement.

Many PwPD are married, just like the rest of the population. I've seen marriages thrive and a few that failed, in part, due to Parkinson's. If you are married, remaining active and engaged in life, as a partner, is essential. The more you fight for your quality of life, the better chance your marriage will have of surviving and thriving going forward. It takes two to make a marriage work. Your diagnosis didn't change that.

If you are single, you may be apprehensive about whether the dating part of your life is over. Not everyone will be willing to get involved with you due to your diagnosis. That just means they weren't the right one. The right partner will not allow Parkinson's to stand in the way of a good thing. Besides, as we age, we are all battling our own health challenges—cancer, diabetes, COPD, or heart conditions. You got Parkinson's.

As long as you stay on top of your condition and are honest with yourself and your partner, there will be far greater things to consider in your dating life. Dating partners may not come right out and express their reservations about your disease. Educate them and show your capabilities through examples of how you live to allay their fears.

Your Battle Plan

1) Are you keeping active socially?

2) Are you sharing your travel needs with your travelling companions?

3) Are you communicating your wants and needs to your loved ones?

4) Which activities do you most want to continue?

28. Read the Label

I am writing this manual like my Parkie brain thinks. I will jump around from here to there and still attempt to have it all make sense to you in the end. This chapter is a good representation of how my mind works.

This morning I was lying in bed, half-asleep. My mind wandered from subject to subject, somewhere between my dream-world and reality, when I realized that I needed to expand upon my "clean diet" comments in this book. Now sure, with today's technology, I could go back and insert it into the previous chapter on diet, and you would be none the wiser. That didn't seem appropriate. These things just pop up, and so that is how I intend to present them to you.

I believe my current clean diet is pertinent information and cannot imagine why it escaped me earlier, since it is a major foundation of my successful journey so far with PD.

While not fully understood or studied enough, it is fairly common knowledge that chemicals, additives, and preservatives in our foods are not good for us.

Unnatural ingredients may not kill us today or cause any issues of immediate concern, yet, they do have a negative impact on our bodies over time. I recently read about the long-term buildup of microplastics in our bodies. I don't think they even know all of the potential issues this may present. Other stories reported that the various pesticides absorbed from fruits and vegetables and the chemicals associated with dry cleaning or household cleaning products may remain in our bodies for an extended time.

With Parkinson's disease, we must limit as many unnatural things from entering our bodies as possible. Some of the chemicals are believed to contribute to our disease, although, not enough research has been done to fully understand these negative effects.

You and I do not have the luxury to wait on years of research. We need to act now, since we already have PD. That's why I choose to stick, as closely as possible, to a diet of foods in their most natural forms.

Unfortunately, the names we assign to various ingredients are too simplistic to explain what we eat every day. The availability of convenient and processed options has literally changed the whole game.

Let's begin with an example of what you can choose

to eat for lunch.

Option One:
Pork, water, sea salt, molasses, onion powder, celery powder, lemon juice, vinegar, cherry powder, garlic powder, onions, cucumbers, celery, soybean oil, egg yolks, paprika

Option Two:
Ham, water, dextrose, salt, sodium phosphates, sodium erythorbate, sodium nitrite, soybean oil, sugar, vinegar, egg yolks, modified cornstarch, mustard flour, paprika, calcium sodium EDTA, lemon juice, cucumbers, xanthan gum, alum, polysorbate 80, turmeric, natural ham flavor, malic acid, citric acid, yeast extract, natural smoke flavor, lactic acid, sodium lactate, red 40

Okay, there you go, which one would you like to eat for lunch? I know I am tired from just typing all of that. The choices above are both labelled "Ham Salad." Yet, their components are immensely different. Which one would you rather consume, to feed your brain and your body? It really does matter. Every little thing we ingest becomes a part of us. Foods are our resource materials we utilize to continue living and thriving.

That was fun. Let's try another one.

Option One:
Potatoes, vegetable oil, maltodextrin, salt, sugar, buttermilk powder, nonfat dry milk, butter, monoglycerides, calcium stearoyl lactate, natural flavor, sodium acid, sodium bisulfate, citric acid, mixed tocopherols

Option Two:
Potatoes, butter, milk, salt, pepper

Both of those options are mashed potatoes. Option One takes four to five minutes in the microwave. Option Two requires peeling and cutting potatoes, dirties a pot, and takes probably twenty minutes of my time. But, in my humble opinion, the second option tastes way better!

We could repeat this exercise over and over. The conclusion for me is that I will always prefer to eat things in their most natural forms. It matters.

I know how much better I feel physically by limiting all of the excess junk from my body. I can and will eat about any food. However, I am consciously selecting healthier versions. I take the time to read labels, and I do not mind taking a few minutes to prepare a more nutritious option. This is something you should try. You will not regret it.

Your Battle Plan

1) What changes can you make to eat healthier?

2) Have you read the labels on your favorite snacks?

3) Can you spend a few extra minutes in the grocery store to read product labels?

4) What's for dinner tonight?

29. Independence

Independence is a topic that will vary from individual to individual. We are all at different ages, different stages, and operating on our own levels. We can be anywhere between total independence and requiring 24/7 assistance. Many of us either have or will need a caregiver to some degree in our future. So, in this chapter, I will describe my own personal situation.

I am quite independent. I live alone with three furry creatures. I do my own laundry, cooking, driving, finances, and yardwork. I realize that I am far from perfect at these things, but I treasure my independence, so I tolerate my imperfections. I have become an impulsive shopper. I get crazy ideas and act upon them, in the spur of the moment. I perform tasks in an illogical manner. I forget far more than I remember. Lots of imperfections. Fortunately, to this point, none have become fatal flaws. I am proactive in recognizing these concerns and seek solutions before they become bigger problems.

Let me provide a few examples. I consciously created new habits to avoid leaving the faucet running in the bathroom or forgetting to turn off the stove burner when I've finished cooking. I am prone to forgetting to move the laundry to the dryer. I developed morning and evening rituals that trigger me to take vitamins and medicines. Fortunately, my furry roommates are quick to remind me if I am tardy with their meals, so that is never a problem.

My specific solutions to these challenges are unimportant because you will develop your own ways to trigger your brain to act. What is effective for me probably won't work for you.

For my shopping impulsiveness, I've employed what I call a "wait a day" strategy. It is not 100% foolproof, but it helps. If I feel I cannot live without an item, I wait a day and see if I still feel the same way. It's amazing how your mind can change in a day.

Now, let's be realistic, if I need milk or toilet paper, I am not going to make myself wait a day. However, there are many nonessential items that I can ponder before purchasing. It limits my impulsive tendencies.

Just yesterday, I encountered an instance of my impulsive shopping tendencies. I receive periodic e-mails from Converse, the shoe company, because I have been a past customer, repeatedly. I owned my first pair of All Star shoes, beginning in either the ninth or tenth grade. I wore that same pair of shoes clear through my senior year in high school. I loved them. Their popularity waned over the years. Recently, they reappeared and are cool again, only now they are called Chuck Taylors. Since high school, people have disparaged my shoes. "Those have no arch support. They're horrible for your feet!" But I only recall how comfortable they always felt. So, I eventually bought me a red pair of Chucks. My memory was accurate. They were tremendously comfortable for me, like walking barefoot.

After about a year, I followed up by adding a green pair. Later, I added a yellow pair. I even got a light blue high-top version. These shoes rarely wear out, so I still have them all! The red ones are showing their age now, probably seven years old, but they still are functional. I wear these sneakers for everyday types of use, plus for exercising and cycling. They get the full experience.

I mentioned that Converse sent me an e-mail. You see, it's early spring here right now, and they just came out with a new color. It's Herby Green! They look so cool! Who could possibly pass up a pair of Herby Greens? Oh my, how I was tempted! I just had to have them! I was gonna be stylin' and the center of attention in those bad boys! But, then I remembered I'm supposed to wait a day. I didn't want to wait a day, but I did. I still *want* those shoes, but I know I certainly do not *need* those shoes. Therefore, I will not buy those shoes. At least not today.

As you can tell, it is a daily battle. My body and brain want to feed those feel-good parts inside of me. Sometimes a new pair of shoes can be one way to accomplish that. It is okay to feed those pleasure centers. Just be careful not to overindulge.

Driving is a very big discussion topic with Parkinson's disease. Many PwPD drive just fine. When the time comes that you don't feel as confident behind the wheel, or others are telling you that you are no longer a safe driver, please err on the side of caution. You do not wish to harm yourself by causing an accident. But more importantly, what if your stubbornness and refusal to give up driving caused injury or death to someone else, possibly a child? Do not risk others' lives.

Freedom is easier to achieve nowadays without being the one behind the wheel. Between friends and family, rideshare services, and other transportation options, you can be on the move. This topic causes a great deal of stress in PD families. If you are facing this obstacle, seek the opinions of your medical team and make an informed and proper decision.

Your Battle Plan

1) What habits or rituals do you need to create to compensate for forgetfulness?

2) What changes do you need to make for your safety or the safety of others?

3) What changes are you being stubborn about accepting?

30. You Are Not Alone

Here in America, approximately 90,000 people are diagnosed with Parkinson's disease each year. Many more are either misdiagnosed or undiagnosed. Worldwide, it is estimated that there are over 8.5 million of us, a number which has doubled in the past twenty-five years. It is definitely a growing problem.

There are many famous individuals who have shared or are currently sharing their PD diagnosis with us—Alan Alda, Muhammad Ali, Neil Diamond, Michael J. Fox, Kirk Gibson, Rev. Billy Graham, Rev. Jesse Jackson, Ozzy Osbourne, Pope John Paul II, and Janet Reno. Several of these public figures did not immediately come forward with their Parkinson's diagnosis. They had the same concerns as you, worried about how others would react and the possible social stigma. A few were forced to reveal their conditions due to bad publicity—falling or tripping in public and being accused of being drunk or on drugs. However, they eventually revealed their conditions to help others.

Muhammad Ali continued to make public appearances and became an inspiration, even lighting the 1996 Olympic flame. And in 1997, the Muhammad Ali Parkinson Center was opened in Phoenix, Arizona.

The person who has done the most for Parkinson's research is activist and actor, Michael J. Fox. The Michael J. Fox Foundation (MJFF) is "dedicated to finding a cure for Parkinson's disease through an aggressively funded research agenda and to ensuring the development of improved therapies for those living with Parkinson's today." MJFF has funded almost $2 billion in research programs as of this book's initial printing date.

A few celebrities were misdiagnosed with Parkinson's before doctors realized their mistakes. Grammy Award winner, singer, and songwriter, Linda Ronstadt, gave an interview after her misdiagnosis to explain she had been forced to give up her singing career. She pivoted and forged ahead, doing speaking tours and writing an autobiography. Her eventual diagnosis was progressive supranuclear palsy.

Peanuts creator and cartoonist, Charles M. Schulz, was initially thought to have Parkinson's disease. His condition was actually essential tremor.

After Robin Williams' tragic death, his wife reported he had been in the early stages of Parkinson's disease. His autopsy indicated diffuse Lewy body dementia. However, in early PD, Lewy bodies are limited in distribution. These apparent discrepancies support the need for more study into PD with dementia versus diffuse Lewy body dementia.

Those are a few famous folks, but most PwPD are much less famous, like you and me. Yet, there are inspirational heroes among us. It is wonderful to see how ordinary people step up and lead by example when it comes to PD. They do not seek fame or special recognition, they work hard to live their best lives. Get involved with your local Parkinson's community. You will encounter these amazing individuals. In time, you might become one yourself.

Do not isolate from the world at large. You have no reason to be embarrassed or ashamed by your circumstances. Most individuals will be quite understanding and even attempt to help you. Get out in the world, and enjoy this life as much as possible, or invite it to come to you. If your situation truly prevents you from going out, then invite friends, family, the kids, the grandkids, or the neighbors over for game night, a bonfire, or to watch the Super Bowl.

Keep engaged with people. Educate people about PD. Share your experience. You don't need to be a Debbie Downer about it.

Explain your condition to help others to feel at ease. This is especially important around kids. Let them see that you are still fun to be around.

Demonstrate your exercises and ask them to try. Keep the experience as positive as possible. Remember that Parkinson's is not only affecting you, but everyone around you as well.

Your Battle Plan

1) Who else do you know with Parkinson's disease?

2) What makes you feel the most insecure about having PD?

3) Are you still getting together with your family and friends?

4) Are you reassuring your family and friends that you are doing okay?

31. Kylee's Story

My take on Young-onset Parkinson's disease?

What a world of questions were in my head, years of feeling and noticing changes about my physical self, what was happening? As symptoms worsened, I noticed I was becoming off-balance. I had a stiff arm and loss of dexterity with my left hand, with spastic arm twitching, an uncontrollable tremor. My left side was dysfunctional and irritable.

Many asked, "How are you? Are you okay?" Some asked, "Why do you look stiff?" Others, not so tactfully asked, "What's wrong with you?" These questions became numbing, in addition to my everyday walk, talk, and dos or don'ts.

My primary doctor told me to walk more, to clear my head. It was then when a sound of a boxing bell, one that ends each round, rang out in my mind. It became my priority to find a team of medical professionals for myself and my wellbeing—a movement disorder neurologist, a massage therapist, chiropractors, and a physical therapist. These weekly appointments and therapies became my need and desire for muscle movement, circulation, and body resensitizing.

On September 5, 2019, I was diagnosed with Parkinson's. I was thirty-nine years old. They called it Young-onset Parkinson's disease. It was mind-challenging. How does one prepare? Parkinson's disease is like a piñata. It's never filled the same and has different strokes for different folks! There are good days and bad days. I thought my years ahead were no longer valuable, but I've learned they can have a renewed purpose.

Diagnosis gave me a new understanding as to why my everyday activities were difficult—like swimming and walking long distance, which cramped my feet and toes. Stressors, good or bad, caused bursts of tremors and twitches. I now could define the reasons why! Over the years, I've retaught myself to confidently ride a bike again, regained confidence to run, and the hardest part of this change was repairing my "old" self and creating my "new" self.

The ongoing challenge is helping myself to learn the "new" me is a daily work in progress. Whether through meditation, mindfulness, therapeutic therapy, or organized workouts, I am fortunate to have found outlets, other PwPD like me, and so many who encourage me to achieve my lifetime milestones.

I am living life again. I am living my best life now.

I am a daughter, sister, wife, mother, friend, and mentor. I am a Rock Steady Boxer, a Rock Steady Head Coach, and a Movement Disorder business owner. I am always working on reshaping my mental and physical health.

Let the world know, ask questions, and find the team that will listen, speak, and challenge you to become a better you. Tomorrow is a new day, it's a restart to your new beginning!

— Kylee Pagán, 44 years old
Owner, Mindful Motivational Movement, Air Force Veteran, Parkinson's Rock Steady Boxer, Certified Rock Steady Head Coach, CPT, YCT

32. Change is Constant

It doesn't matter whether you have Parkinson's disease or not, change is going to happen. That's life. We do not all like or enjoy change. We tend to resist it as we age. Part of the reason is that it becomes more challenging for us to learn new skills or different ways of doing things.

I am reminded of my grandfather when I think about adapting to change. He was born in 1900 and passed away in 1986. That man experienced some serious changes, and he was not particularly a fan of any of them. I was around to witness a few very old ways of doing things, thanks to him.

On his farm, we put up hay loose, not in bales, with a team of horses that pulled a large wooden sled. He mowed weeds with a scythe and trimmed with a sickle. We plowed gardens with a horse-drawn plow. He didn't own a television and never installed indoor plumbing. If it was too cold to go to the outhouse, then we would use the bucket on the stairs that led from the living room up to the bedroom. The house had no central heating or air conditioning. Water was hand-pumped from a well in the side yard. He was only on an Interstate highway once in his life, for probably less than ten miles, and he was terrified. I actually do not know that he ever traveled 100 miles from where he grew up.

Toward the latter part of his time, he was begrudgingly forced to embrace certain modern advancements. We did get a tractor, and a neighbor had a hay baler that made the small square bales, and we switched to doing the hay that way.

Despite not owning a television himself, he would watch it sometimes if he was at our house. I think he kinda liked it, but would never admit to it. He believed many technological advancements promoted laziness and kept people from working hard.

By the 1980s, such things as microwave ovens and edgier rock and roll music meant that he had become a man out of his time. He truly struggled to understand the modern world in which he lived.

Now, at sixty-one years old, I am far enough along to have witnessed many changes of my own. I began in my grandfather's world. Now, I live among the Internet and self-driving automobiles, I even understand that flying taxis are almost a reality. My climate-controlled house is filled with gadgets operated by simple voice commands. My car beeps at me when I weave out of my lane or approach an object too quickly. Just about anything imaginable is delivered to my doorstep within a matter of hours. I drink water from a bottle and eat foods I hadn't even heard of thirty years ago. The changes are absolutely incredible and ongoing.

I do not need to embrace every change, but I open myself to the ones that can enhance my life and my experience. This becomes more essential with having Parkinson's. My short-term memory, my mobility, my ability for social interactions, and a bunch of other things can and will be altered as time marches on.

The voice assistant in my home is invaluable. She provides me information, such as news and weather. I ask her to set timers, alarms, and reminders. She entertains me and my cats with music. Other features I may need later are controls for lights or a home alarm system that calls for help.

Eventually, I might utilize a cane, a walker, or even a wheelchair. These potentialities are not unique to Parkinson's, but they are perhaps more prevalent concerns regarding our futures. I've heard too many stories of PwPD being stubborn about using these aids. Unfortunately, you place yourself in danger if you're not helping yourself. Who cares what it looks like? It is better than falling and causing a life-altering injury. I'd choose bruised pride over a broken hip every time.

A great exercise program will greatly reduce these dangers. My coaches teach me how to fall properly to minimize injury. Yet, there still may be a time when each of us would be wise to use these types of devices. We cannot allow foolish pride to stand in the way of a better quality of life. I already have a bed rail, so I don't roll out of bed during my vivid dreaming. I wear funny-looking socks that spread out my toes, to combat toe curling. I wear a dental appliance for sleep apnea. When the neuropathy in my hands flares up, I slip on wrist splints. I can be quite a sight as I head off to bed. It's all okay. These medical devices make my days better.

There will be additional changes in my future, of that I am certain. I can mourn, feel sorry for myself, get angry, be a mean and grumpy old man, or I can utilize the best solutions available and keep going. That's what I choose to do, what I can control. That is the way life works. It's a bumpy ride at times. Changes keep coming. Work with what you have and make the most of it.

Battle Plan

1) What changes have you witnessed in your lifetime?

2) How do you react to change?

3) Which modern technology or gadget would you find most helpful?

4) Are you stubborn about retaining your independence?

33. Planning Ahead

This chapter touches on a topic that most people wish to put off for as long as possible. However, you should not avoid it. In fact, this moment in life is a wake-up call and reminder to get your affairs in order. If you haven't already, you should create a will, a healthcare directive, and assign a legal power of attorney, in case the need arises. You may even want to consider the benefits of setting up a trust for your assets. An attorney can draw up these legal documents for you. Legal documents make things much easier for your loved ones in the future.

You may wish to preplan your funeral and burial wishes. Even though you might not require these services for decades, you should set a plan. It can always be amended later.

Do you have life insurance? Parkinson's will exclude you from certain policies but not all. The same is true with health insurance. You may have limited choices. A qualified insurance professional can walk you through the options available to you.

Substantive conversations about your possible future should be a part of planning with your family.

Who will be a caregiver if needed? Are you going to a facility or moving in with a family member? Discussing these matters ahead of time can make the transitions easier. Knowing who will care for you or even your pets can be a big relief. Don't turn these future arrangements into a mystery for your loved ones to solve.

Your Battle Plan

1) Do you have your own affairs in order?

2) Do you need to set up a trust or assign beneficiaries to financial accounts?

3) Do you need to review your current insurance and health care policies?

PART IV
FORTIFYING YOUR ARSENAL

I have spent much of my energy in the previous chapters attempting to relay my viewpoints on matters that are relevant to a more generalized Parkinson's audience. People are diagnosed with Parkinson's disease in different stages of life and with symptoms which can be so wide-ranging, it is a challenge to address the myriad of ways that the disease could impact you.

In this part of the book, I will discuss other weapons to consider adding to your arsenal. While each of the following chapters may not apply directly to you, hopefully, they can provide something of value to be useful in your journey.

34. Caregivers

I realize that readers of this book may be loved ones or caregivers of those of us who have been diagnosed with Parkinson's disease. First, let me say, may God bless you for sticking by us and being there during what can be an extremely stressful experience. Unfortunately, not everyone has your courage. I've witnessed spouses, significant others, and family members who walk or run away. They either cannot or choose not to stay and take on the additional burdens which may lie ahead. You, however, are attempting to educate yourself about this coming battle. A million times, thank you!

I warn you that your particular loved one may be unwilling or unable to express their gratitude. They may not be fully aware that it is you giving them a nudge forward or the support they need to keep going. They might be mad at the world, thinking, "Why me?" They may be in denial that they are in need of your help. Often, being a caregiver is a thankless job. But, I am here to tell you that I know you are invaluable and you are appreciated by me and others like me. The things you will be called upon to do, simply out of love, are not easy.

Your loved one may be facing the fear of losing independence, losing their dignity, and losing their ability to do the activities they have always enjoyed. They may not respond well to you telling them they can no longer be the captain of their own vessel.

You will be required to practice extreme patience and immense understanding during this experience. Be careful not to become your loved one's taskmaster. As long as they have their mental faculties about them, do not unilaterally make decisions without including them in the process. This is still their life. Even if it takes a bit longer, work together to develop solutions and compromises. Help them to be on board with changes involving their care. If they are battling you *plus* battling the disease, then they may feel like a cornered animal. That's not a good way to feel. Try to take this on with as much love and patience as you can muster.

Depending how advanced the PD is, a caregiver will play different roles. You can be an active advocate playing a key role in slowing the progression and maintaining quality of life for the PwPD.

I've talked about the huge benefits of vigorous exercise for Parkinson's. Well, one of the best motivators to get your loved one moving is for you to exercise with them! Yes, that's right. I just threw you under the bus and told you that you need to get your butt moving too! Not only will it help your PwPD, it will be a healthy activity for you.

Previously, I mentioned I attend exercise classes specifically for PwPD at Rock Steady Boxing. Friends, wives, husbands, daughters, sons, sisters, brothers, girlfriends, boyfriends, and even an occasional grandchild will work out alongside their loved ones. I believe it inspires the PwPD to work harder. They can feel the love. If a member's PD is farther along, the partner will often serve as a personal assistant during these gym sessions.

You can be the cheerleader who encourages your person to keep living. Help them find solutions to obstacles that arise. Encourage them to travel or go places for as long as possible. Suggest things such as a cane, or if they require additional assistance, a walker with a collapsible seat, or a wheelchair for longer outings. Help arrange breaks or rest times, so they can recover and rejuvenate during these adventures. Don't be impatient or frustrated with them for taking breaks. Be a partner in problem solving. Motivate them to stay active.

Coordinate activities. Give your loved one a purpose, something meaningful to do. When preparing dinner, include them in meal prep. Don't leave them to sit idly watching television. Ask them to read instructions, mix the ingredients, or hunt for that colander that you cannot seem to locate. I understand these tasks need to be tailored to your loved one's current abilities, but keep them involved.

After dinner, pull out a board game, a deck of cards, or a jigsaw puzzle. Games can provide hours of entertainment while exercising the mind. I like the brain teaser puzzle books I find in stores and online. Work on those together. Maybe you both enjoy painting, playing music, or dancing. Yes, PwPD can dance from a wheelchair.

Be silly, be creative. Fill your loved one's life with laughter and activities. Do not allow them to space out in front of a television or a cell phone screen for most of the day. Sure, we all enjoy television or online videos, but keep them engaged the majority of the time.

If your PwPD requires significant care assistance, please make time for yourself. Do not lose *you* in their disease. Arrange for others to be your stand-in periodically, so that you can have the energy to enjoy your own activities or have time to decompress. Do not feel guilty. If you do not take care of yourself, you will be absolutely no use to anyone else either.

Depending on the severity of their disease, they might qualify for in-home assistance. Aside from any help you may receive from family and friends, there are organizations that specialize in giving a family caregiver a break. Some are operated through federal and state governments, others through privately operated companies. Investigate these resources through your local Area Agency on Aging or a similar organization. Inquire about a local caregiving company and programs available in your area. Social workers at hospitals can serve as informational resources too, along with your own doctors and therapists.

In my area, there are support groups specifically for Parkinson's caregivers. Seek out opportunities in your area. If there isn't a support group already, then you or another caregiver you know would be a good candidate to start one.

I realize I have hinted at some doom and gloom in this chapter. However, your experience with Parkinson's won't necessarily be horrible. I've just been trying to cover a few of the possible outcomes. The truth remains that the more proactive your loved one is in their care, the more likely they will live a long life and pass away from some unrelated illness, just like anyone else. This disease is not always the end of the world. It's just a new chapter that requires adjustments, and you can play a huge role in your loved one's success.

Your Battle Plan

1) Which exercise activities can you do regularly with your PwPD?

2) Do you need to purchase some new board games or puzzles?

3) What activities can you do for yourself?

35. Service Animals

Are you aware that there are service animals for Parkinson's disease? Yes, it is true. They are trained to assist with various activities of daily living. Service dogs can enhance your balance while you walk and provide specific support when climbing stairs. These functions reduce the likelihood of falls. They are trained to recognize freezing and provide a nudge to encourage movement in the frozen leg. They can assist you with getting in and out of chairs. These animals can fetch many items such as canes, medicine bottles, remote controls, and clothing items. They can be taught to speed dial 9-1-1 in an emergency.

Owning a service dog has a few extra side benefits as well. It encourages the PwPD to exercise more because the dog must go outside and be fed and watered. A dog is also a loving companion and will help minimize loneliness or feelings of isolation.

Of course, a service dog is an added expense to your budget. Food, vet bills, and other miscellaneous costs are not insignificant. Additionally, you must be dedicated to caring properly for and loving the animal who is giving all that they have to you. It must be a reciprocal relationship.

If cost is a concern, there are nonprofit groups that you can find online that provide service animals to those with disabilities, at a reduced cost or for free, for individuals who qualify.

Your Battle Plan

1) Which activities of daily living are currently most challenging?

2) Would you benefit from a service animal?

3) If so, why not begin investigating this option today?

36. The War

War is waged through a long series of battles. We have covered several of those battle scenarios throughout this book. We have identified weapons we can use to fight these various foes. Now, let's look at the bigger picture.

As wonderfully magnificent as life may be, we already know that it will come to an end one day. That is a predetermined outcome. The most we can truly hope for is to have a long, quality journey through this incredible experience. We are fortunate to even exist in the first place. It is nothing short of miraculous.

We will all face our own unique battles. Some face poverty, hunger, physical handicaps, and disabilities. Others live in areas torn apart by wars. Many will develop heart disease, cancer, fibromyalgia, COPD, or have a stroke. Heck, I could go on all day listing the various ailments people face. While life is definitely a blessing, it does come with struggles. In our case, one of these struggles happens to be Parkinson's disease.

So, in the big picture, what is your goal with Parkinson's? Your goal is probably similar to mine. I hope to live as full and complete of a life as possible and die in my sleep at a ripe old age from something that happened in an instant, no long-term suffering and no pain. That's a perfect scenario, isn't it? Short of that ideal ending, let's examine what we can control.

We cannot control yesterday. It is gone. We can attempt to rewrite the history to our liking, but whatever happened in the past, that's not going to change now. We cannot do much about tomorrow either. Our only ways to impact tomorrow are to plan for what we believe might occur and to prepare by doing the most we can do today.

In my experience, if I attempted to predict my future, I'd often be wrong. Unexpected events alter our future plans. Just look at PD. Did you have a plan for life with Parkinson's? I know I didn't. So, in the end, all we can really, truly control is today, this exact moment in time. That is where the past ends and the future begins. You control your actions right now in the present.

With any war, being able to adapt to changing conditions and circumstances and making frequent adjustments is a great advantage. The slower you are to pivot, the better opportunity you offer to your enemy to gain the upper hand.

Parkinson's disease is definitely a powerful enemy,

and we need to remain vigilant in our fight every single day. We need to be aware of subtle changes in our conditions and be quick to address new symptoms. This disease will continually probe our defenses for weaknesses and exploit them to gain an advantage.

In order for us to reach that ripe old age, with a quality life we are seeking, we cannot allow PD to ever gain an advantage without an all-out fight. Complacency is not an option.

During my own walk with PD, I have dealt with episodes of nerve pain which at times were quite severe. Those episodes definitely interfered with my daily quality of life. There was one period where I basically lived on a sofa, in constant pain, for three months. Multiple tests and procedures were performed until we determined what alleviated my pain. Then, the goal became to not only cure the acute problem, but to minimize its frequency and likelihood of recurrence. This was accomplished through a combination of medications, medical therapies, and strengthening exercises. It took about a year to achieve what I would call full healing. Now, I only experience occasional minor chronic flare-ups. Understanding how to manage these symptoms enabled me to take control, so that they no longer ruled my life.

Here is another episode from my own history. I developed a strange blurring in my vision. It happened randomly. My primary care doctor and my neurologist didn't have answers. They referred me to a specialist who quickly identified the problem as an ocular migraine.

The best way I can describe the condition is as if someone put an oily substance over my eye lens. I can see light and colors, but my vision is severely impacted. These experiences last approximately twenty to thirty minutes at a time. Fortunately, they are painless, but they leave me unable to function because I literally cannot see. That's why the diagnosis of a type of migraine seemed odd to me. Now, I have a name for it and methods for minimizing it. I am told that spasming in my eye muscles, associated with Parkinson's, is probably to blame.

I am going to offer one more odd example. I went to a dentist for a filling. My mouth was numb. They proceeded to work. It was going well, and I experienced no pain. Then, my leg began to quiver. Over the passing minutes, the quiver became a shake. Soon, both legs were shaking, and eventually reached the level of such a violent shake that the dentist had to pause the procedure for a half an hour, as I shook uncontrollably.

Once this subsided, the dentist completed her work and fixed the tooth. She advised me going forward to always ask for numbing injections without epinephrine in them. Apparently, I had become hypersensitive to what is commonly referred to as "epi." I didn't connect the dots until sometime later when I was having a conversation with other PwPD. We realized that a very large percentage of us experienced the exact same issue when receiving numbing injections. This was a surprising revelation to us all.

Since then, I've had a couple of dental implants, due to a racquetball incident, and a couple of deep scale cleanings where I requested no epinephrine, and there were no complications. Being proactive and not accepting these adverse reactions as normal, I've maintained a great quality of life.

You may not be able to win every battle in this war. Between Parkinson's, normal aging, and any other health issues you are fighting, your body will change over time. But, fight every step of the way to ensure your best quality of living. This war will probably not end quickly, since there is no cure. Our best defense is to weaken the control Parkinson's attempts to gain over us. The benefits of each battle you win will pay dividends for a long time to come. I see it in my own life and in the lives of the many people I know with Parkinson's. Not only is it beneficial to them, but also to their families and friends who surround them. We are here on Earth to live, not to sit idly by and wither away. So, let's not allow this enemy to prevent us from making the most of our lives. Let's fight and win against Parkinson's disease every day.

37. You Can Do This

Virtually none of us expected to be in this position. Parkinson's disease simply showed up one day as an uninvited guest. Unfortunately, without a current cure, it is a permanent guest for the remainder of our lives. Yes, there are multiple stages of grief to be processed with this diagnosis. It is natural to mourn for a while, feel self-pity for a while, be angry for a while, and even live in denial for a while. But do not get stuck in any of those stages of grief. Eventually, you must accept that this is your new reality.

Once you have accepted this fact, then you can move forward, discovering the best ways to battle this enemy. I hope this book and its battle plan questions will help you to accomplish that. I hope you learn, as I have, that this isn't the end. You have worthwhile adventures ahead of you. Your original plan might be altered, but it can still be a high quality life.

I understand that I seem overly positive to some. But I believe in my heart that if you could witness just a fraction of what I have seen, you would feel the same way too. That's why I wrote this book. I felt compelled to share my experiences and my hope for a quality future. I want you thriving, not just existing. Strive to reach goals you never thought possible. Show Parkinson's disease that *you* are in control.

Commit to trying new things you didn't think were still possible. Display the courage to keep moving and growing. Become a living example for those who will be diagnosed in the future, to show them the way to lead a good life with Parkinson's disease.

Lastly, I want to hear from you. I want you to let me know how you are doing and how you are winning this battle one day at a time. You can do this! I know you can!

Resources

National Institute of Neurological Disorders and Stroke
www.ninds.nih.gov

Parkinson's Foundation
www.parkinson.org

The Michael J. Fox Foundation for Parkinson's Research
www.michaeljfox.org

Davis Phinney Foundation for Parkinson's
www.davisphinneyfoundation.org

Rock Steady Boxing
www.rocksteadyboxing.org

LSVT Global — LSVT BIG and LSVT LOUD
www.lsvtglobal.com

American Parkinson Disease Association
www.apdaparkinson.org

Dance for PD, A Program of Mark Morris Dance Group
www.danceforparkinsons.org

Brian Grant Foundation
www.briangrant.org

PWR! Parkinson Wellness Recovery
www.pwr4life.org

ADA — U.S. Department of Justice, Civil Rights Division
www.ada.gov

Acknowledgements

I could write an entire book just thanking all of the people who have taken part in making my life with Parkinson's disease a successful journey. But, here are a few who deserve special mention.

Meng Yan, Ph.D., Indiana University, thank you for facilitating my becoming a guest lecturer and for your strong encouragement for me to write this book.

Coach Kristy Rose Follmar ACSM, CPT, CIFT, you are a rock star! Former World Champion Professional Boxer, one of the foundational pillars upon which this Parkinson's exercise movement is built, an inspiration to countless others, and most importantly, you are my dear friend. I am so honored that you took the time to contribute the foreword to this book. You will forever be one of my favorite people in the whole world.

My Rock Steady Boxing coaches and staff, thank you for all of your hard work and dedication and for putting up with my shenanigans. You've made a world of difference whether you realize it or not.

Suzanne Purewal, more than just the publisher, the chief editor, my guide and mentor, as well and my friend and confidant, thank you for encouraging me to make this book the best it could be. Without your hard work and dedication, I could not have accomplished writing this book.

Douglas Bland, we just work well together, don't we? Whether it's exercising or goofing off, we match. You enhance my life on a regular basis. I want to thank you as well for contributing your story. We are on this Parkinson's ride together, and I'm blessed to call you my friend.

Doreen Fatula, my eccentric, positive, boxing and karaoke partner, we need more of you in the world. Such a good human. Thanks for sharing your words about your life with PD. I'm very lucky to have your input in these pages and to have you as my friend.

Steve Gilbert, you have such a quiet and gentle spirit, and you lead by example. Your life since diagnosis has been nothing short of remarkable. You are probably my biggest PD hero. I look up to you as a marker of what I hope to be someday. I am also extremely grateful that you agreed to include your story in these pages. I cannot say thank you enough.

Kylee Pagãn, my very dear friend, my karaoke buddy, my fellow PwPD, and my inspiration, thank you for contributing your story. You and I share a unique connection. I don't really know how to put it into words, but you know exactly what I mean.

Cathy Delaney, we've seen a lot together, haven't we? Thanks for the valuable information I needed to include in these pages. You rock!

Kimberly Jacobson, thank you so much for volunteering to pre-edit my manuscript and for the invaluable feedback. It's people like you who make me look good.

About the Author

L. E. Hewitt has had an established career as a professional musician, business owner, and author. Diagnosed with Parkinson's disease in 2015, he found himself on a new and unexpected life path. It was an uncertain future at first, but with education and experience came knowledge and understanding. Combining his previous experience as a published author and the many years of living with Parkinson's, he realized that he had an important message to offer to others who may be facing this or similar diagnoses. There are numerous resources available from the perspective of the medical community, but this book is designed to be a guide from the perspective of the patient.

The author currently resides in Indiana where he enjoys his life as a parent and grandparent, along with being active in the Parkinson's community, both locally and nationally. He is fortunate to be surrounded by a highly qualified and skilled staff of experts and an eclectic cast of characters who help him to maintain a very good quality of life.

L. E. Hewitt loves to hear from his readers!

If you enjoyed this book,
please leave a review on Amazon, Goodreads, or
L. E. Hewitt's Facebook Author Page!

Check out the latest news and events on his website:
www.lehewitt.online

Printed in the USA
CPSIA information can be obtained
at www.ICGtesting.com
CBHW060935010924
13781CB00058B/973

9 781732 288041